Fundamentals of Health Care Improvement

A Guide to Improving Your Patients' Care

Second Edition

Gregory S. Ogrinc, M.D., M.S.

Linda A. Headrick, M.D., M.S.

Shirley M. Moore, R.N., Ph.D.

Amy J. Barton, R.N., Ph.D.

Mary A. Dolansky, R.N., Ph.D.

Wendy S. Madigosky, M.D., M.S.P.H.

Forewords by
Maureen Bisognano
and
Paul Batalden, M.D.

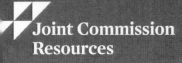

Joint Commission Resources

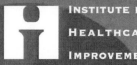

INSTITUTE FOR
HEALTHCARE
IMPROVEMENT

Senior Editor: Katie Byrne
Senior Project Manager: Cheryl Firestone
Project Manager: Andrew Bernotas

Manager, Publications: Lisa Abel
Associate Director, Production: Johanna Harris
Executive Director: Catherine Chopp Hinckley, Ph.D.

Joint Commission/JCR/JCI Reviewers: Lisa Abel, Kimberly Anderson-Drevs, Caroline Christensen, Linda Faber, Linda Hanold, Catherine Hinckley, Tanya Huehns, Cynthia Leslie, Mondher Letaief, Deborah Nadzam, Sharon Sprenger, and Susan Whitehurst

Institute for Healthcare Improvement (IHI) Reviewers: Jane Roessner and Val Weber

Joint Commission Resources Mission

The mission of Joint Commission Resources (JCR) is to continuously improve the safety and quality of health care in the United States and in the international community through the provision of education, publications, consultation, and evaluation services.

Joint Commission Resources educational programs and publications support, but are separate from, the accreditation activities of The Joint Commission. Attendees at Joint Commission Resources educational programs and purchasers of Joint Commission Resources publications receive no special consideration or treatment in, or confidential information about, the accreditation process.

The inclusion of an organization name, product, or service in a Joint Commission Resources publication should not be construed as an endorsement of such organization, product, or service, nor is failure to include an organization name, product, or service to be construed as disapproval.

This publication is designed to provide accurate and authoritative information in regard to the subject matter covered. Every attempt has been made to ensure accuracy at the time of publication; however, please note that laws, regulations, and standards are subject to change. Please also note that some of the examples in this publication are specific to the laws and regulations of the locality of the facility. The information and examples in this publication are provided with the understanding that the publisher is not engaged in providing medical, legal, or other professional advice. If any such assistance is desired, the services of a competent professional person should be sought.

Joint Commission Resources, Inc. (JCR), a not-for-profit affiliate of The Joint Commission, has been designated by The Joint Commission to publish publications and multimedia products. JCR reproduces and distributes these materials under license from The Joint Commission.

The Institute for Healthcare Improvement (IHI) is an independent not-for-profit organization that works with health care providers and leaders throughout the world to achieve safe and effective health care. IHI focuses on motivating and building the will for change, identifying and testing new models of care in partnership with both patients and health care professionals, and ensuring the broadest possible adoption of best practices and effective innovations.

Printed in the U.S.A. 5 4 3 2 1

Requests for permission to make copies of any part of this work should be mailed to
Permissions Editor
Department of Publications
Joint Commission Resources
One Renaissance Boulevard
Oakbrook Terrace, Illinois 60181 U.S.A.
permissions@jcrinc.com

ISBN: 978-1-59940-569-8
Library of Congress Control Number: 2011942130
For more information about Joint Commission Resources, please visit http://www.jcrinc.com.

To Karen, Nick, Andy, and Peter, for your love and encouragement. To Linda Headrick and Paul Batalden, for your continual guidance and support.

—G.S.O.

For Duncan Neuhauser and Paul Batalden, exceptional teachers of health care improvement. For David and Daniel Setzer, the heart of my life.

—L.A.H.

To the "Summer Camp" group who have nurtured my thinking and passion about health care quality and safety for many years.

—S.M.M.

For JoAn Gocsik, R.N., my mom and mentor, for teaching me patients always come first.

—A.J.B.

To the next generation of health care providers inspired to continually improve.

—M.A.D.

For my students and their future patients; with gratitude to my husband, Craig, and children, Isaac and Sarah, for their support—and patience!

—W.S.M.

Contents

Foreword *to the second edition*

My sister asked me three questions, and I had no answers to them. These questions led me on a journey to think about how to improve the health care system. Although I was a staff nurse in an intensive care unit at the time, I began to see a new responsibility when I looked at the system through my sister's eyes. The responsibility to care for patients was familiar and rewarding, but I saw a new challenge: How could I improve the systems of care to ensure safer, more effective care?

The journey started when Robbie was just a few months old. Robbie was the first grandchild in my large family and was a happy, healthy, and adored child. When he was two months old, Robbie went to his pediatrician for his well-baby checkup; after declaring him in perfect health, his doctor advised my sister that he was going to administer Robbie's vaccinations. Shortly after returning home, Robbie was very ill, and my sister took him back to the pediatrician's office. He was transferred to an academic medical center and admitted to the ICU in respiratory distress. After a week in the hospital, Robbie was well enough to come home to his family, and he recovered completely over the following weeks.

At Robbie's four-month check up, his doctor again told my sister that Robbie was in great health. As he proceeded to prepare the routine vaccination dose, my sister reminded him of what had happened after the two-month vaccination. The doctor paused and told my sister that Robbie's previous illness had not been a reaction to the vaccine. Despite her challenges, he assured her that Robbie would be fine but that he would administer only half the dose. He administered the vaccination, and Robbie died within 24 hours.

The questions my sister asked that changed my career were these: (1) How could the office and hospital patient records be so separated that the doctor couldn't see Robbie's whole journey? (2) How could the doctor not have known that a half dose was the wrong treatment? and (3) Why didn't he listen to me?

These questions bring to the surface some of the problems in our health system today. Good practitioners struggle with broken systems and processes. Atul Gawande, a surgeon and best-selling author, has calculated that a physician interacting with a patient today has more than 13,000 possible diagnostic options and can prescribe from over 6,000 different medications. The complex journey of care requires new skills for all of us. It requires that we know how to, and do, deliver the best evidence-based care in accordance with an individual patient's circumstances and preferences and that we work cross-professionally to make the care system safer.

This book is your guide to becoming a complete health care professional, a strong caregiver, and an effective improver. The examples you'll study will be familiar, but the approaches to improvement may surprise you. By the end, you'll see the health care world with new eyes. You'll see systems in addition to symptoms. You'll think in daily PDSA cycles for improvement in addition to major change initiatives. And you'll see a new role for every health care professional.

Our patients rely on us to connect the pieces of the journey and to make it as safe as it can be. They rely on us to design and work within systems of evidence and with the knowledge supports we need. And they need us to listen.

Just five years ago, when I was teaching quality improvement methods to third-year medical students, I was rebuffed and heckled. "We have no power," they said. "Go call the CEO if you want things to improve." They recounted the challenges in their work with frustration and helplessness in their voices. They saw the problems in their daily work but saw no way out of the daily process failures. It's different today. In the few years since that depressing class, medical students, nursing students, and health professions students are building new skills in addition to the profession-specific knowledge they gain during their learning years. They know, now, not just what care to deliver but also how to improve the systems in which they deliver that care. Just three years ago, the Institute for Healthcare Improvement opened the IHI Open School for Health Professions (http://www.IHI.org/IHIOpenSchool)—a new way for students to build these crucial skills and to collaborate with other learners worldwide to improve care.

Here's an example of what makes me so optimistic today. Recently, three medical students met online through the IHI Open School virtual community and aligned their schedules to spend a month at IHI. They came and learned with our staff, met with experts from around the world, and began to improve safety in their earliest days of learning. They met Atul Gawande and studied operating room safety. They used WIHI—IHI's "radio station"—to teach fellow medical students throughout the world how to use surgical checklists. They collaborated to write a peer-reviewed article, "Check a Box. Save a Life: How Student Leadership Is Shaking Up Health Care and Driving a Revolution in Patient Safety" (http://www.ihi.org/offerings/ihiopenschool/resources/Pages/Publications/CheckaBoxSaveaLifeStudentLeadershipDrivingPatientSafety.aspx), and they developed an iPhone app to download the WHO Surgical Safety Checklist. These students have learned what you will learn in this book. You'll build a new way to see health care, from the patient to the system. You'll see the problems more clearly, and you'll see how to eliminate them. The skills you will build as you work through *Fundamentals of Health Care Improvement* will make you a better clinician, a more valued team member, and will enrich your career as you serve the patients who rely on us for excellence.

Maureen Bisognano
President and Chief Executive Officer
Institute for Healthcare Improvement

Foreword *to the first edition*

This book is about a better future: better outcomes for individual patients and populations of health care beneficiaries, better health care system performance, and better health care professional development—all linked together and in the lives of the people who will become tomorrow's doctors.

These doctors and their fellow young health professionals will:

- Know that to be a professional and to be recognized as one, work will always have two aims: "to do your job and to improve your job."
- Be more than the naive system players of earlier times—they will know that every system is perfectly designed to get the results it gets—and that, therefore, their job goes beyond protecting their patients *from* the systems in which they work to being responsible for the design and redesign of those systems.
- Know that to achieve any sense of personal professional mastery, they must be involved in changing and improving the systems in which they work.
- Understand how measurement can be a friend of learning, redesign, and professional mastery and not just a tool for auditors, researchers, and payers.

This book is for them . . . and for those who seek to enable their futures. The basic knowledge and skills in this book can become the means of restoring a sense of "agency" in the health professionals of tomorrow. These skills will move advocacy into changed practices. Further, they will know that as professionals, they can use the systems they design and redesign to minimize the burden of illness—and from that knowledge will come a sense of mastery that will be deeply attractive.

Competence for a professional is always about knowing "that" something is so and knowing "how" something comes to be. Professional work is about performance: knowledge-in-action to meet the human need you face. In medicine, it is the interweaving of the science of disease biology and the science of clinical practice. Learning that interweaving and the professional work that flows from it is largely a matter of experiential learning—learning from doing and reflecting on it. This book is about that.

New information systems will enable a very different health care system. Information systems need accompanying process and system changes to make anything different occur. To do so will require attention to the material that is introduced in this book. This is likely to be a dynamic process, better considered in "verb forms" than in static "noun forms." Life in this world will be made more sensible by the topics introduced in this book.

These new professionals and their enabling faculty will enjoy the springboard from this book as together they will learn the lessons—the lessons that can only come by practicing and reflecting on that practice. Knowledge and skill for the redesign of care can come from the users of this book—learners and their teachers—actually engaging in tests of improvement and learning from them; but all improvement practice is practice, and to learn from it requires reflective review on the practice and its patterns.

Parker Palmer thinks that good teaching and learning often involve creating "space" within an idea, creating some working boundaries around the topic, and offering hospitality for the journey of discovery. Let your use of this book help you create that space for reflection, improvement, and learning.

The good news is that early signs show that professionals in the next generation of health care know they need to learn the material in this book and know they need to develop some skills in the application of the knowledge involved. They have seen the frustrations of those who have preceded them in the profession—frustrations about the prospect and reality of changing the practice and the context in which they work. Those in this new generation have grown up aware that the context for living is a world constantly re-creating itself. They want to take action on the gaps that can be seen. They value the agility that rapid-cycle tests of change rest on. This book and its tools and approaches can help them and their teachers together as this learning proceeds.

The authority of the authors of this book derives, in part, from their own generative "authoring" work in improving the quality of their own health care–giving and from what they have done to foster diverse learning environments that enable others to learn. In short, this book offers a great opportunity to learn, to practice, and to become a leader in tomorrow's health care system. Enjoy it.

Paul Batalden, M.D.
Professor of Pediatrics,
Community and Family Medicine Director,
Center for Leadership and Improvement
The Dartmouth Institute for Health Policy and Clinical Practice
Dartmouth Medical School

Introduction

Fundamentals of Health Care Improvement: A Guide to Improving Your Patients' Care, Second Edition, will help students of the health care professions diagnose, measure, analyze, change, and lead systems improvement in health care. By applying knowledge and skills you have acquired throughout your medical and nursing courses of study and training, you will learn how to effectively shape and create reliable, high-quality systems of care for your patients.

Chapter 1: The Gap Between What We Know and What We Do

Chapter 1 explains the concept of a quality gap and describes ways in which health care can be improved through analysis of the quality gap. Various models are presented to further emphasize the importance of identifying gaps in health care and continuously working to improve patient care.

Chapter 2: Finding Scientific Evidence to Apply for Clinical Improvement

In Chapter 2 you'll learn steps to take when collecting and evaluating evidence for the improvement of care. You will gain a clear understanding of the following: how to find evidence on the basis of a properly formulated question, how to evaluate the quality of evidence and research, and how to identify the most appropriate resources to use in finding evidence.

Chapter 3: Working in Interprofessional Teams for the Improvement of Patient Care

Chapter 3 describes the positive outcomes that arise from productive teamwork and provides a set of criteria for identifying effective teamwork. In addition to learning how to assess factors that affect the way teams function, you'll learn how to create a team comprising members from multiple health care professions.

Chapter 4: Targeting an Improvement Effort

Chapter 4 offers valuable information on getting started with effective improvement work. After reading this chapter, you will be able to identify and focus on areas that need improvement. In addition, you will be able to organize your improvement goals by writing a clear aim statement.

Chapter 5: Process Literacy

In Chapter 5 you will learn the importance of describing the process of care as well as steps for choosing the most appropriate method for communicating about the process. Also included are instructions for considering the organizational culture and context features that influence clinical processes. After reading this chapter, you will understand how to create a process model that is understandable to everyone who is part of the care team.

Chapter 6: Measurement Part 1: Data Analysis for Improvement

Chapter 6 emphasizes the necessity of using data to improve health care and explains that different types of data are used to support different objectives. This chapter also discusses using a balanced set of measures for improvement work and introduces the clinical value compass, a tool for identifying measures.

Chapter 7: Measurement Part 2: Using Run Charts and Statistical Process Control Charts to Gain Insight into Systems

In Chapter 7 we discuss the benefits of analyzing data over time so that you can monitor the changes that occur in a system. Common cause variation and special cause variation are compared and contrasted in detail to provide an overview of what types of variation might be expected in a system. Examples of run charts and statistical process control charts help you understand the importance and benefits of displaying data over time.

Chapter 8: Understanding and Making Changes in a System

Chapter 8 will help you manage complex system change and will show you how to identify barriers to change. In addition, complex adaptive systems are defined and described in a list of eight principles. The Plan–Do–Study–Act method is introduced to illustrate the testing and assessing of small cycles of change.

Chapter 9: Spreading Improvements

Chapter 9 will enable you to identify strategies for sustaining and spreading change. As you read the practical, three-step approach for planning a successful spread effort, you will also learn how to overcome barriers to successful spread.

Chapter 10: A Chapter for Educators: Designing Ways for Students to Learn to Improve Care

Serving as a guide for educators, Chapter 10 discusses the five stages of skill development in health care professionals and how to cultivate competency through practice-based learning and improvement. The chapter also offers educators five principles to consider when building educational experiences in health care improvement.

IHI Open School Resources

The IHI Open School offers 16 online courses, free to students and health professionals, in quality improvement, patient safety, leadership, patient- and family-centered care, and more. See http://www.ihi.org/offerings/IHIOpenSchool/Courses.

In addition, the Open School offers a range of resources, free to all, including videos, case studies, podcasts, featured articles, chapter activities, and more. See http://www.ihi.org/offerings/IHIOpenSchool/resources.

Acknowledgments

The authors wish to acknowledge the time and effort of the following people:

- Lisa B. McAllister, administrative assistant for the Office of Research and Innovation in Medical Education at Dartmouth Medical School, for her work securing copyright permissions.
- Rebecca S. Graves, reference librarian at the University of Missouri Health Sciences Library, for her contributions to Chapter 2.
- Pat Busick, M.S., C.I.A., Iowa Lutheran Hospital, and Julie Gibbons, R.N., B.S.N., C.I.C., Iowa Health Des Moines, for their willingness to share their story with us and for their contributions to Chapter 9.
- Tina Foster, M.D., M.P.H., M.S., and Leslie Hall, M.D., for their contributions to the development of Chapter 10.
- Paul Batalden, M.D., for providing an insightful review and an inspirational Foreword to the first edition.

In addition, Joint Commission Resources gratefully acknowledges the author team for the time, talents, and dedication each member wove into the second edition of this book. Special thanks to Maureen Bisognano, president and chief executive officer of the Institute for Healthcare Improvement, for her graceful and thought-provoking Foreword to this edition.

CHAPTER 1

The Gap Between What We Know and What We Do

OBJECTIVES

After reading this chapter, you will be able to do the following:
1. Identify gaps in the quality of health care.
2. Recognize the difference between making decisions for one patient's care and making decisions for a system of care.
3. Describe how the Model for Improvement is used to help close the quality gap.

"Every system is perfectly designed to get the results it gets."—Paul Batalden, M.D.

Olivia Baddour is a 65-year-old female who comes to the emergency department with a complaint of chest pain. Over the weekend, while working in her garden, she experienced several episodes of chest tightness, pain, and shortness of breath. Each of these episodes resolved itself, but this morning she had a much longer, more severe episode while carrying groceries up the stairs. The symptoms today were accompanied by cold sweats and aching arms. She called 911 and was taken to the emergency department at Northeast Regional Medical Center.

In the emergency department, Olivia is cold and sweaty, and she appears ill. On physical exam, her lungs are clear to auscultation, and her heart has a regular rate and rhythm with a normal S1 and S2—no murmurs, gallops, or rubs. Her abdomen is flat and nontender. She has normal bowel sounds. There is no edema in her ankles. Josephine Lyons, the emergency department physician, continues her assessment.

Diagnosing a Health System That Is Ill

For a straightforward case such as Olivia's, most clinicians are comfortable identifying the major components of the history and physical exam. We also could identify additional elements:

- What is the patient's family history?
- Is she a smoker?

- Has she had a workup for chest pain in the past?
- Does she have high blood pressure?
- What is her pulse rate?
- Does she have jugular venous distention?

After reviewing the history and physical exam, a clinician might consider that this patient is experiencing an asthma attack, a heart attack, pneumonia, or perhaps gastroesophageal reflux. Many clinicians could identify diagnostic testing that should be done: an electrocardiogram, a chest x-ray, and likely some blood work.

In the scenario above, Olivia is, in fact, having a heart attack—also called a myocardial infarction (MI). Josephine, the physician, proceeds to treatment options: administering an aspirin, oxygen, and a beta-blocker (medicine to slow down the heart rate, lower blood pressure, and decrease the work of the heart). Depending on the location and capacity of the hospital, the physician might also arrange for the patient to have coronary angiography and angioplasty, with placement of a stent to open up her coronary artery. Another option would be to administer medications to break up the blood clot.

In just a few paragraphs, we comfortably review the history, physical exam, workup, and treatment for the acute stages of an individual patient experiencing an MI. This is how we are trained in medical school and nursing school. We evaluate and treat *individual* patients. In many ways, determining when a patient is ill is straightforward. We use knowledge and multiple skills: Take a history, perform a physical and psychosocial exam, review diagnostic tests, confer with other health care professionals, and synthesize large amounts of data in order to provide evidence-based care for patients. It is more challenging to determine when a health care *system* is ill. Health professions students are not routinely taught how to assess, diagnose, and treat systems in health care. Think about this important question: How can you change systems so that you can apply the best evidence for the improvement of patient care?

This book will help you, as a learner, diagnose, measure, analyze, change, and lead system improvement in health care.

This book will help you, as a learner, diagnose, measure, analyze, change, and lead system improvement in health care. It provides the foundation of knowledge and skills specific to health care system improvement as well as exercises to develop these skills. Improving health care is a skill-based activity. In many ways, learning and practicing these skills requires effort that is similar to learning and practicing diagnostic and treatment skills; however, instead of an individual patient focus, the focus is on creating reliable systems of care that produce the highest quality for every patient, every time.

Finding the Quality Gap

Examining outcomes of care is one way to identify when and where a system is broken. Let's focus on the use of beta-blockers as a treatment for acute myocardial infarction (AMI) and see if we can diagnose areas where the system is not working well. Figure 1-1a on page 4 shows data about the percentage of beta-blocker use after an AMI. These are data from a research study that used a U.S. Medicare database (one considered very solid for research).* Published in 2000, the study compares outcomes of care for major teaching, minor teaching, and nonteaching hospitals.[1] The hospitals are stratified by number of resident physicians and number of hospital beds.

One conclusion of the study was that major teaching hospitals provided better-quality care than did minor and nonteaching hospitals. As shown in Figure 1-1a, nonteaching hospitals prescribed beta-blockers 36% of the time, minor teaching hospitals 40% of the time, and major teaching hospitals about 49% of the time. While it is true (according to this study) that major teaching hospitals may provide better-quality care than minor and nonteaching hospitals do (these differences were statistically significant), the authors of the study note another important conclusion in their discussion: In the year 2000, patients such as Olivia Baddour were receiving beta-blockers only 49% of the time *at best*.[1] Because beta-blockers are inexpensive, effective, and well tolerated, good-quality care dictates that the rate of usage should be at least 95%—and probably closer to 100%. This difference between 49% and 95% is called the *quality gap* (*see* Figure 1-1b on page 4). The quality gap is the difference between the expected level of care (95% beta-blocker usage) and the measured outcomes of a system (49%). These gaps in quality exist in all specialties and at all levels of the health care system.

Although this is a clear illustration of a quality gap, this study was published in 2000, using data from the late 1990s. Even though this specific quality gap has largely been closed in the United States, why was there such a large gap in 2000? The 2000 study by Allison et al. uses Medicare* data from the entire United States, so perhaps a snapshot of the system at a local level would give a different picture of how the system is performing.[1] With this in mind, let's examine Figure 1-2 on page 5. The data in this figure are more recent (2009) and more local (although anonymous). We can assess beta-blocker usage on several levels: Hospital 1 in 2009, Hospital 2 in 2009, and the primary care Pine Tree Clinic's patients in 2009. It is also possible to compare local performance to the top 10% in the United States and to the national average. These local systems (that is, at the hospital level and clinic team level) were performing better in 2009 than were the systems in the 2000 study (*see* Figure 1-1a). Why is this? Perhaps these hospitals and individual clinicians improved their skills over that period? Can we be sure that the quality gap that we recognized in 2000 is related to the systems of care and not just to clinician knowledge? Is there a way we can improve (diagnose and treat) the system so that each patient gets the best care every time?

One possible explanation for the differences in beta-blocker use shown in Figures 1-1a, 1-1b, and 1-2 is that the scientific data were not sufficient in 2000, and thus

---

* Medicare is the U.S. federal health insurance plan that includes most individuals age 65 and older.

FIGURE 1-1. *Percentage of Beta-Blocker Usage for Medicare Patients Diagnosed with an Acute Myocardial Infarction (AMI), Stratified by Teaching Status of the Hospital*

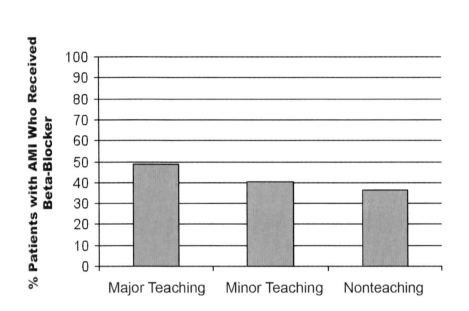

Figure 1-1a. The percentage of beta-blocker usage for Medicare patients diagnosed with an AMI is stratified by teaching status of the hospital.

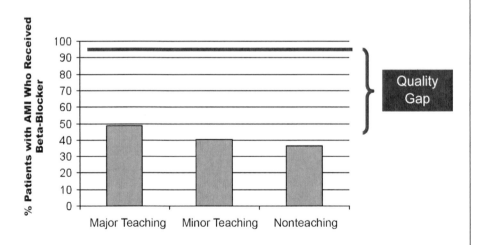

Figure 1-1b. This chart shows the quality gap between where the system is performing and where it should be performing.

Source: Allison J.J., et al.: Quality of care at teaching and nonteaching hospitals. *JAMA* 284:2994–2995, Dec. 2000. Copyright © 2000 American Medical Association. All rights reserved.

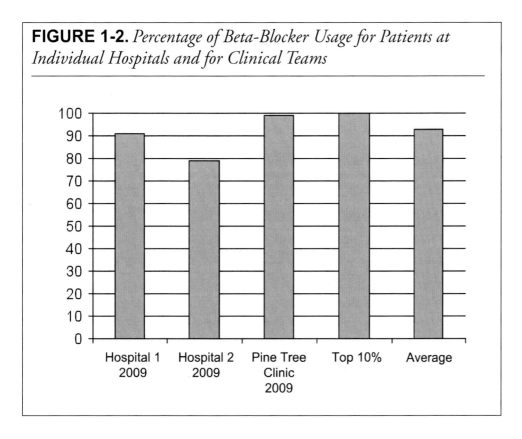

FIGURE 1-2. *Percentage of Beta-Blocker Usage for Patients at Individual Hospitals and for Clinical Teams*

clinicians were not aware that using beta-blockers was the right treatment. Perhaps more scientific evidence was needed to convince clinicians that beta-blockers are an appropriate medicine to administer after MI? As mentioned earlier, there are several undeniable conclusions about beta-blockers and MIs: They reduce mortality, are inexpensive, and are tolerated well. Data gleaned from a review of articles (considered very strong evidence that has been summarized from many clinical trials) supporting beta-blocker use after MIs have been available since 1984.[2–5] Thus it is even more surprising that more than 50% of patients with AMI were *not* receiving these medications in 2000—16 years later! Surely electronic means of accessing information makes the dissemination of evidence-based practice easier in 2011, but the evidence alone is insufficient to change and improve systems of care.

Evidence-Based Improvement

There is much more to putting evidence into practice than just having the right research evidence. The right evidence is often the focal point of most health professionals' education. Figure 1-3 on page 6 is a model that shows the components of evidence-based improvement.[6] This model demonstrates how the best scientific evidence can be combined with knowledge of an individual system to produce improved outcomes for patients. The right-hand side shows that what we desire for our patients is *measured performance improvement*—for each individual patient and for our populations of patients. We want high-quality care for our patients in many domains: clinical, functional, satisfaction, and cost. We often start (on the left side of Figure 1-3) with *generalizable scientific evidence*. Generalizable scientific evidence comes from health care research in which investigators control for context and build knowledge that is generalizable across many contexts. This is where research design, carefully constructed methodology, and statistical analyses are used to evaluate treatments and therapies to determine the extent to which they are effective. As shown in the earlier beta-blocker example, 16 years after evidence of the effectiveness of beta-blockers was known and widely disseminated in review articles, the treatment of patients with beta-blockers still lagged behind—even at academic medical centers.

The Missing Connector

What's missing in health care is a connector—a set of knowledge and skills to take the best evidence and put it into practice consistently and reliably for the improvement of care for patients. The connector must take into account the local context of the system being improved so that the people, the existing processes, and the structure of the system are understood. The people, processes, patterns, and structures are different between Hospital 1 and Hospital 2 in Figure 1-2; therefore, the analysis of the system and the changes to improve the outcome will be different between Hospitals 1 and 2. The evidence about beta-blockers is the same, but the systems in which to incorporate that evidence are different. To improve care for patients, it's necessary to find the best evidence (in this case, that beta-blockers reduce mortality and morbidity after MI) and link that evidence of best care with the specific knowledge of the local system in which that care is being provided (for example, use of computerized order entry, location of hospital, presence of an integrated cardiology unit).

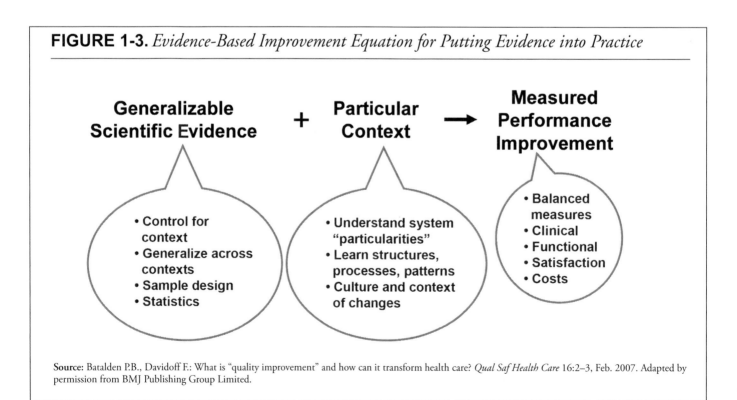

FIGURE 1-3. *Evidence-Based Improvement Equation for Putting Evidence into Practice*

Generalizable Scientific Evidence

+

Particular Context

→

Measured Performance Improvement

- Control for context
- Generalize across contexts
- Sample design
- Statistics

- Understand system "particularities"
- Learn structures, processes, patterns
- Culture and context of changes

- Balanced measures
- Clinical
- Functional
- Satisfaction
- Costs

Source: Batalden P.B., Davidoff F.: What is "quality improvement" and how can it transform health care? *Qual Saf Health Care* 16:2–3, Feb. 2007. Adapted by permission from BMJ Publishing Group Limited.

Caring for the System

Just as there are standard methods for assessing, diagnosing, and treating individual patients, an analogous set of tools exists for diagnosing and treating systems of care (*see* Table 1-1 below). For an individual patient, the clinician starts with a history and moves to a physical exam and diagnostic tests before arriving at a set of recommendations for therapy: comfort measures, medications, surgical interventions. Similarly, someone within a system (for example, a clinician such as yourself) often notices, through his or her own experience in the system or from discussions with others, that the system is not working well. Rather than just be frustrated by the system, clinicians can go on to the next phase of diagnosing the system: creating process flow diagrams, reviewing outcomes data, or creating fishbone diagrams. Finally, with a diagnosis and understanding of the system, the improvement team can recommend and test changes. Caring for a system is a natural extension of the skills that are used to care for individual patients.

Caring for a system is a natural extension of the skills that are used to care for individual patients.

Describing Improvement

The right-hand column in Table 1-1 describes the process of improvement in health care. In the past, there have been many terms (and many acronyms) used to describe improvement in health care: quality management (QM), total quality management (TQM), continuous quality improvement (CQI), systems-based practice (SBP), and practice-based learning and improvement (PBLI), to name a few. While each of these has nuances and roles in specific situations (for example, compliance, resident physician training, nursing education), we favor the more generic *quality improvement* and, even more simply, *improvement*, which incorporate aspects of many of these.

TABLE 1-1.
Comparison of Diagnosing and Treating an Individual Patient Versus Analyzing and Improving the System of Health Care

	Individual Patient	**System of Health Care**
Initial Workup	• Chart review • History • Physical examination	• Individual experience in the system • Feedback from others in the system
Further Workup	• Blood work • Laboratory tests • Radiographs • Functional tests	• Observation of the process • Process flow diagrams • Cause-and-effect diagrams • Outcomes data
Therapy/ Treatment	• Pain management • Surgical intervention • Medications • Watchful waiting	• Model for improvement • Root cause analysis • Plan–Do–Study–Act cycle

DEFINED:
Quality Improvement

Quality improvement is best defined as "the combined and unceasing efforts of everyone—healthcare professionals, patients and their families, researchers, payers, planners and educators—to make the changes that will lead to better patient outcomes (health), better system performance (care) and better professional development (learning)."

Quality improvement is a shared responsibility.

Quality improvement is best defined as "the combined and unceasing efforts of everyone—healthcare professionals, patients and their families, researchers, payers, planners and educators—to make the changes that will lead to better patient outcomes (health), better system performance (care) and better professional development (learning)."[6(p.2)] This definition captures the focus of the three pillars of improvement (*see* Figure 1-4 below)—on health outcomes for patients, on performance of the health care system, and on the development of health care professionals. The inclusion of "everyone" in the center is key. Including everyone in this manner can have profound implications for an organization. For example, Walt Disney World, in Orlando, Florida, has a reputation for being impeccably neat and tidy; guests expect it to be so. A Disney executive, when asked how many people are on the cleanup crew, answered, "over 45,000." He was not referring to an army of custodians, but to each and every person on the Disney payroll. Keeping the parks tidy is a priority for every person who works there. Similarly, the improvement of outcomes, systems, and professional development are foci for quality improvement for everyone from a new student to a practicing unit nurse to resident physicians, attending physicians, and chief nursing officers. Quality improvement is a shared responsibility.

FIGURE 1-4. *The Batalden and Davidoff "Triangle Diagram" to Demonstrate the Relationship of Everyone to the Three Core Pillars of Quality Improvement*

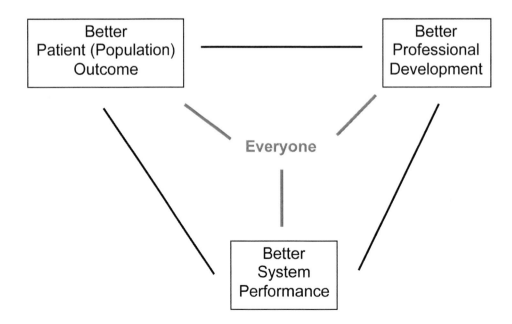

Source: Batalden P.B., Davidoff F.: What is "quality improvement" and how can it transform health care? *Qual Saf Health Care* 16:2–3, Feb. 2007. Adapted by permission from BMJ Publishing Group Limited.

Relationships Among the Pillars

How are the pillars of the triangle diagram shown in Figure 1-4 related to one another? Consider an example of two leaders in an academic medical center. One leader, the vice president for nursing, has an advanced nursing degree and a master's degree in business administration. The other leader is the senior associate dean for education at the medical school and holds a medical degree. The vice president lives in the systems performance world, and her feet are firmly planted on the "better system performance" pillar. The education dean's feet are firmly planted on the "better professional development" pillar. Each of these individuals must recognize that the decisions and changes they recommend to the care system (or to the educational system) will also affect the other two pillars. In other words, even though his or her feet are planted on one of the pillars, the eyes and ears must recognize their close proximity to the other two pillars. The improvement of care is interdependent on each of these elements. As a learner in the system, you also are a vital part of each of these pillars, and your efforts to improve the system of care will influence all of them.

Thus, improvement is the professional responsibility of everyone in the health care system—and it depends on much more than just having the right scientific evidence at hand. Fortunately, a model exists that demonstrates effective ways to connect our best-practice evidence with our local health care delivery system. The Model for Improvement (*see* Figure 1-5 on page 10) provides a structure for diagnosing and treating systems of care.[7] The following is an introduction to the model and a brief example of its use. We'll use this model throughout this book and return to it often as we delve deeper into the specific knowledge and skill components of clinical improvement.

The Model for Improvement

How do we know the Model for Improvement is effective? There are many examples in the literature of systems that have been improved with the methods proposed in this model. This methodology has been used to improve coronary artery bypass grafting surgery,[8] assess and improve cost and staff satisfaction on a general internal medicine inpatient unit,[9] improve care for patients in a multispecialty spine center,[10] and reduce falls and injury from falls in hospitalized patients.[11] Each of these represents an example of improving the system of care for patients. Across these examples there is one very consistent bottom line: *Improving health care is a contact sport—it is something that we* do. Improvement does *not* occur by simply attending a lecture, sitting in a meeting, reading a book (not even this book!), or performing online simulations. It is achieved through experience in applying these methods, and this experience is necessary for achieving competence in the full range of skills needed for clinical practice.

FIGURE 1-5. *The Model for Improvement*

What are we trying to accomplish?

How will we know that a change is an improvement?

What changes can we make that will result in improvement?

Act | Plan

Study | Do

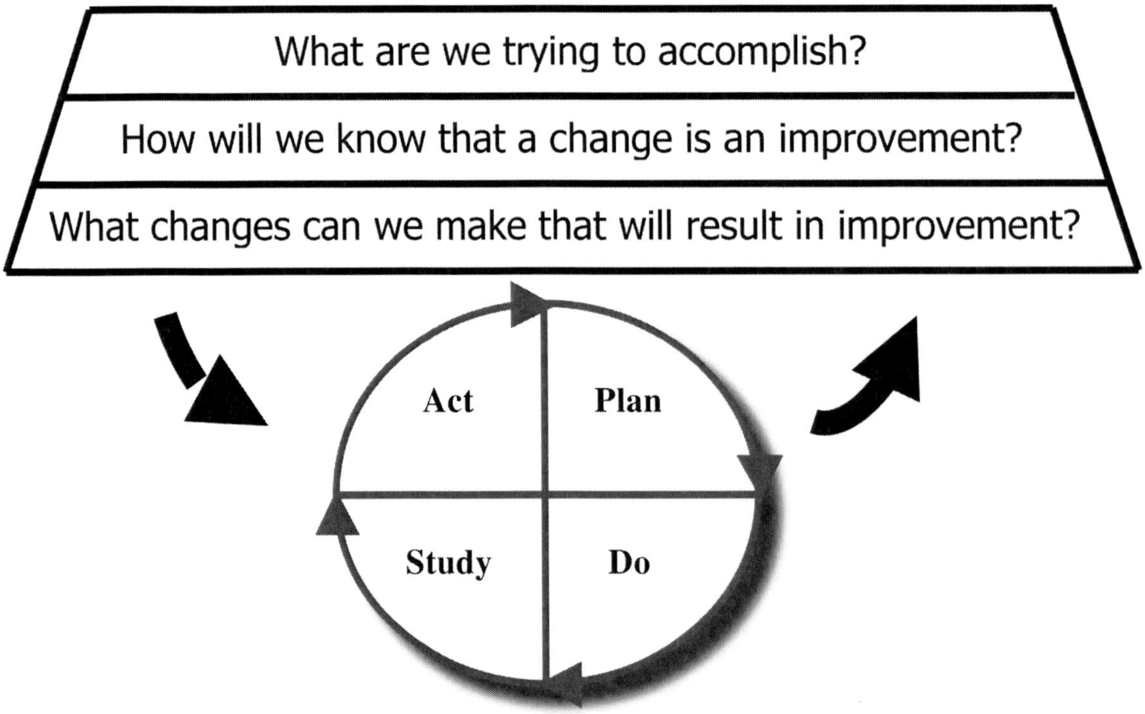

Source: Langley G.J., et al.: *The Improvement Guide: A Practical Approach to Enhancing Organizational Performance,* 2nd ed. San Francisco: Jossey-Bass, 2009. Printed with permission.

Three Questions in the Model for Improvement

If system improvement is a skill to learn and practice, how is it done? In this book, we focus on the Model for Improvement because it is widely used and easily available. The model distills the improvement process into three questions:

- What are we trying to accomplish (aim)?
- How will we know a change is an improvement (measures)?
- What changes can we make that will result in improvement (changes)?

Once the answers to these three questions are determined, the Plan–Do–Study–Act (PDSA) cycle is used to design and test changes on a small scale. In this book, we will cover each of these steps in depth in subsequent chapters.

As an introduction to using the Model for Improvement to close a quality gap, let's return to the example of beta-blockers. In Figure 1-2 on page 5, we see a beta-blocker quality gap of over 20%. In Hospital 2 the leadership has formed a team to work on closing this beta-blocker quality gap. The beta-blocker after myocardial infarction (BAMI) team consists of the chief cardiology resident, a cardiac care nurse with training in quality improvement, a medical student, a pharmacist, and the nurse discharge coordinator.

Creating the aim. The BAMI team at Hospital 2 starts by creating an aim:

> "In the next six months, we will increase the rate of beta-blocker usage in patients at discharge after MI to greater than 90%."

This is a strong, clear aim. It reads like the byline from a newspaper article. It states who is going to be working on this aim, what they are going to be doing, what the exact goal is, and when the results should be achieved.

Determining the measures. After setting the aim, the BAMI team determines the measures it will use in judging the success of achieving the aim. For this example, the measure is relatively straightforward:

> "The percentage of MI patients who receive a beta-blocker at discharge from the hospital"

Because this is the same indicator that showed the gap in quality, monitoring this indicator (percentage of patients receiving beta-blockers) monthly will help determine whether progress is being made.

Testing changes. For possible changes, the BAMI team holds a brainstorming session to list how to change the system and ensure that every patient with MI reliably receives a beta-blocker upon discharge. As shown in Figure 1-6 on page 12, the team is able to identify several possible interventions, including the following:

- Educate the physicians about the benefits of beta-blockers.
- Have the pharmacist review medications at discharge.
- Teach the patient and the family that beta-blockers are important to keep the heart healthy.

The BAMI team does not know which of these would be most effective, but by systematically trying each one (using the PDSA methodology), the team can test each intervention and measure its impact.

This brief example oversimplifies the improvement process; in truth, the aim, measures, and changes may take several weeks or months for the team to develop. Care delivery systems do not improve by chance; nor do they improve simply through the development of new knowledge. As indicated in the beta-blocker example, it took almost 20 years for knowledge about the benefits of beta-blockers to become embedded in health care systems and thus close the quality gap (*see* Figures 1-1 and 1-2 on pages 4 and 5); quality improvement can accelerate the system changes needed to close those gaps.

FIGURE 1-6. *The Beta-Blocker After Myocardial Infarction (BAMI) Improvement Team Worksheet*

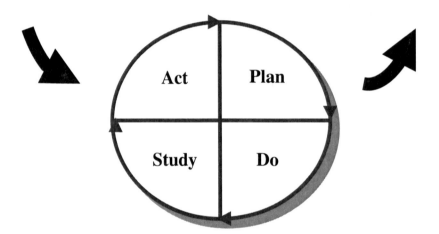

In the next six months, increase the rate of beta-blocker usage in patients at discharge after a myocardial infarction to greater than 90%.

Measure the percentage of patients who have a myocardial infarction and who receive a beta-blocker at discharge from the hospital.

Possible interventions: (1) Educate the physicians, (2) educate the patient and family, (3) have pharmacists review discharge meds, (4) encourage nurses to identify beta-blockers at discharge, and (5) generate prescription for beta-blocker automatically and place it on the patient's chart.

Act　Plan

Study　Do

Source: Adapted from Langley G.J., et al.: *The Improvement Guide: A Practical Approach to Enhancing Organizational Performance*, 2nd ed. San Francisco: Jossey-Bass, 2009. Printed with permission.

Summary

Quality gaps exist in all areas of health care: vaccination rates for children, treatment for patients with posttraumatic stress disorder, surgical wound infections, turnaround time for specimens sent to a pathology lab, follow-up of radiology tests, outpatient blood pressure control, and so on. Quality gaps affect every health care profession, every practice specialty, and potentially every patient. As health care professionals, we have a duty to improve the systems in which we work. Just as you learn to take a history, perform patient assessments and physical exams, and recommend and implement treatments for patients, you also must learn how to analyze and measure systems of care and recommend and implement system-level changes (*see* Table 1-1 on page 7). Our job as health care professionals is not only to *provide* care but also to *improve* care.

Although this may seem a daunting task, the skills for improving patient care systems can be learned like the skills for providing pain management, drawing blood samples, auscultating the heart, or evaluating chest x-rays. This book walks you through the development of improvement skills. It shows you how to evaluate systems and apply changes to improve the delivery of care. This book will give you knowledge to view the clinical setting differently—through a "systems lens." After reading this book, you'll be able to identify how to measure clinical care in a comprehensive way that accounts for clinical outcomes, patient functional ability, patient and staff satisfaction, and even the costs of care. As clinical improvement becomes a routine part of clinical care, you'll be ready to recommend changes to systems that are embedded in the care system so that patients like Olivia Baddour reliably receive the right care at the right time.

References

1. Allison J.J., et al.: Relationship of hospital teaching status with quality of care and mortality for Medicare patients with acute MI. *JAMA* 284:1256–1262, Sep. 13, 2000.
2. Hjalmarson A.: Early intervention with a beta-blocking drug after acute myocardial infarction. *Am J Cardiol* 54:11E–13E, Dec. 21, 1984.
3. Frishman W.H., Ruggio J., Furberg C.: Use of beta-adrenergic blocking agents after myocardial infarction. *Postgrad Med* 78:40–46, 49–53, Dec. 1985.
4. Davenport J., Whittaker K.: Secondary prevention in elderly survivors of heart attacks. *Am Fam Physician* 38:216–224, Jul. 1988.
5. Hjalmarson A.: International beta-blocker review in acute and postmyocardial infarction. *Am J Cardiol* 61:26B–29B, Jan. 29, 1988.
6. Batalden P.B., Davidoff F.: What is "quality improvement" and how can it transform healthcare? *Qual Saf Health Care* 16:2–3, Feb. 2007.
7. Langley G.J., et al.: *The Improvement Guide: A Practical Approach to Enhancing Organizational Performance*, 2nd ed. San Francisco: Jossey-Bass, 2009.
8. O'Connor G.T., et al.: A regional intervention to improve the hospital mortality associated with coronary artery bypass graft surgery. *JAMA* 275:841–846, Mar. 20, 1996.
9. Curley C., McEachern J.E., Speroff T.: A firm trial of interdisciplinary rounds on the inpatient medical wards: An intervention designed using continuous quality improvement. *Med Care* 36(Suppl. 8):AS4–AS12, Aug. 1998.
10. Weinstein J.N., et al.: Designing an ambulatory clinical practice for outcomes improvement: From vision to reality—The Spine Center at Dartmouth-Hitchcock, year one. *Qual Manag Health Care* 8:1–20, Winter 2000.
11. Neily J., et al.: One-year follow-up after a collaborative breakthrough series on reducing falls and fall-related injuries. *Jt Comm J Qual Patient Saf* 31:275–285, May 2005.

CHAPTER 2

Finding Scientific Evidence to Apply for Clinical Improvement

OBJECTIVES

After reading this chapter, you will be able to do the following:

1. Describe the link between the best evidence and the context of care.
2. Recognize the range and depth of questions that should be asked to find supporting evidence for the improvement of care.
3. Recognize the relative strength of research evidence and the difference between filtered and unfiltered evidence.
4. Identify the proper use of resources—including electronic resources and reference librarians—to find evidence for health care improvement.

A team of students from medicine, pharmacy, and nursing is awaiting the start of interprofessional rounds on a medical ward. As they wait, the students comment on today's cold winter weather and on the number of patients admitted with community-acquired pneumonia (CAP).

For the past two weeks, the attending has recommended that the team use a combination of ceftriaxone and azithromycin for empirical antibiotic treatment of CAP. Today there is a new attending, however, who insists that patients receive single coverage with levofloxacin. The new attending is adamant in stating that single antibiotic coverage is simple, appropriate, and evidence based.

The students are confused. Why is the treatment protocol changing? Is it based on the individual preference of the new attending, or does evidence exist to support this approach? During lunch, the students agree to meet at the library after their clinical shift to explore the evidence for treatment of CAP. As they scan the National Guideline Clearinghouse Web site (http://www.guideline.gov), the students come across the section on CAP. This section includes several links to practice guidelines and position statements from many professional organizations, including the American Academy of Home Care Physicians, the Infectious Diseases Society of America, and the Scottish Intercollegiate Guidelines Network.

National Guideline Clearinghouse
http://www.guideline.gov

Each student chooses a different link to research the inpatient care of CAP. The pharmacy student chooses the Infectious Diseases Society of America link and finds that it contains extensive, exhaustively cited information. She has neither the time nor the inclination to read it all, so she moves to the table of summary recommendations. She is a bit surprised to find that empirical treatment for CAP is acceptable with either a combination of third-generation cephalosporin (for example, ceftriaxone) and an advanced macrolide (for example, azithromycin) or with a single agent such as a fluoroquinolone (for example, levofloxacin). When she relays this information to the nursing and medical students, they, too, are puzzled and even a bit dismayed. The students understand the microbiology and pharmacology behind either the antibiotic combination or the individual antibiotic as acceptable empirical coverage for likely causes of CAP; however, these guidelines are confusing to them.

With something as straightforward as antibiotics for a common infection, how is one to decide which is the right recommendation to follow? Both of these recommendations are supported by reams of research, but is one more correct than the other? Can both be right?

The Importance of Evidence-Based Practice

The emphasis on the use of evidence in health care has grown logarithmically in recent years. New scientific knowledge is generated at a rate of more than 10,000 articles per year. The amount and the configuration of data and information can be overwhelming. Since the notion and use of evidence-based practice (EBP) for clinical decision making became prominent in the 1990s,[1–5] the discipline of managing and using evidence has continued to grow.

EBP is defined as "the process of shared decision making between practitioner, patient, and others significant to them based on research evidence, the patient's experience and preferences, clinical expertise or know-how, and other available robust sources of information."[6(p.57)] At the University of Colorado Hospital, this definition of EBP has evolved into health professionals' practice of placing the patient at the center of the practice model, surrounded by sources of evidence and supported by organizational infrastructure (*see* Figure 2-1 on page 17).[7] At the core of the Colorado Patient-Centered Interprofessional Evidence-Based Practice Model is the patient and his or her preferences, values, and experiences. Valid and current research provides the best evidence for the situation.

Sources Beyond Research

When research evidence is limited or inconclusive, the Colorado Patient-Centered Interprofessional Evidence-Based Practice Model identifies eight additional sources of evidence to help inform care:

1. Pathophysiology
2. Retrospective or concurrent medical record review
3. Quality improvement and risk data
4. International, national, and local standards

DEFINED: EBP

Evidence-based practice (EBP) is defined as "the process of shared decision making between practitioner, patient, and others significant to them based on research evidence, the patient's experience and preferences, clinical expertise or know-how, and other available robust sources of information."

FIGURE 2-1. *The Colorado Patient-Centered Interprofessional Evidence-Based Practice Model University of Colorado Hospital © 2009*

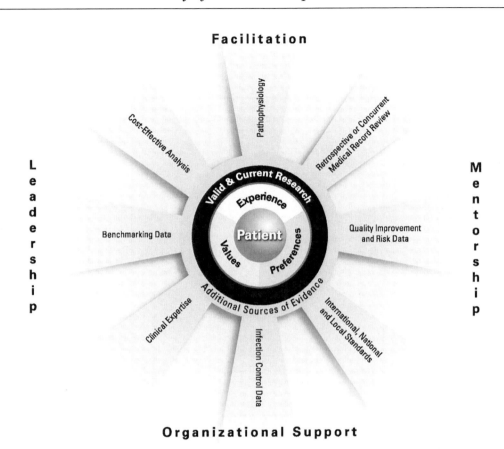

Source: Goode C.J., et al.: The Colorado Patient-Centered Interprofessional Evidence-Based Practice Model: A framework for transformation. *Worldviews Evid Based Nurs* 8:96–105, Dec. 6, 2010. Reprinted with permission.

5. Infection control data
6. Clinical expertise
7. Benchmarking data
8. Cost-effectiveness analysis

EBP involves applying the best-known evidence, using the clinician's judgment, for an individual patient at a point in time. None of these sources of evidence is considered more important than another, although a particular decision may give more weight to one element than to another. For example, a patient who is a Jehovah's Witness may meet all the criteria for a red blood cell transfusion; however, because of the patient's preferences, no blood products would be given. True application of EBP involves bringing patient preferences, experience, and values, along with valid research and additional sources of evidence, to bear on patient care decisions.

EBP involves applying the best-known evidence, using the clinician's judgment, for an individual patient at a point in time.

Limitations of EBP

Over the past several years, EBP has begun to show some of its limitations in its methodological ability to improve care and outcomes for patients. Because there is an abundance of evidence available, finding evidence is usually not an issue. In the example of beta-blocker prescribing after myocardial infarction in Chapter 1, we saw that while strong evidence had been readily available in the published literature for more than 16 years, the data had not made a full impact on practice (fewer than 50% of patients received this treatment). As the students in the opening vignette of this chapter learned, we are awash in evidence that has been packaged into guidelines and reviews. Not all diagnostic and therapeutic situations are backed by evidence, but for those that are (for example, treatment of diabetes, timing of perioperative antibiotics, prenatal testing), application of the evidence in practice is irregular and inconsistent.

Linking of evidence to systems of care. One challenge is that while guidelines are explicit, the application of this knowledge locally is implicit and tacit.[8] Simply making the knowledge available does not bridge the gaps in care.[9] The EBP emphasis on applying evidence to one patient at a time limits its impact by not reliably applying evidence to all patients in a specific system or context. EBP provides a solid foundation for asking the right questions and finding answers to apply to patient care; however, it is limited in scope because it does not explicitly address linking evidence to the systems of care.

Applying the best care to a system is an extension of the precepts and foundations of EBP. Consider for a moment the evidence-based improvement equation introduced in Chapter 1 (*see* Figure 2-2 on page 19).[10] Generalizable scientific evidence is at the forefront of this equation and forms the foundation of improvement. Strong experimental design and sound data analysis are vitally important to build new, generalizable scientific knowledge. Equally important is applying that evidence to a system of care and understanding the local context of care. An assumption is often made that creating the right evidence will lead to improved patient outcomes; however, the transfer of knowledge from scientific evidence to practice and improved outcomes does not reliably occur just from the strength of evidence. So *finding* the right evidence and *applying* that evidence in practice are two separate steps. We need changes in systems of care to apply evidence consistently and reliably. In the Colorado Patient-Centered Interprofessional Evidence-Based Practice Model, the clinical environment in which care is provided (which includes organizational support, mentoring, facilitation, and leadership) is an important contextual factor in the use of evidence. This chapter focuses on finding the right evidence to improve systems.

EBP provides a solid foundation for asking the right questions and finding answers to apply to patient care; however, it is limited in scope because it does not explicitly address linking evidence to the systems of care.

So finding the right evidence and applying that evidence in practice are two separate steps.

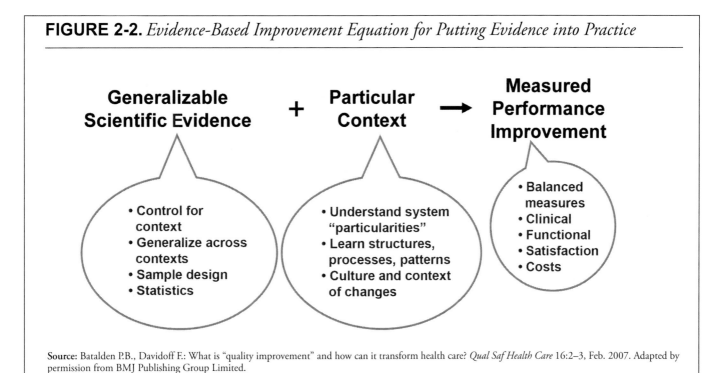

FIGURE 2-2. *Evidence-Based Improvement Equation for Putting Evidence into Practice*

Source: Batalden P.B., Davidoff F.: What is "quality improvement" and how can it transform health care? *Qual Saf Health Care* 16:2–3, Feb. 2007. Adapted by permission from BMJ Publishing Group Limited.

Formulating the Right Question

Finding the right evidence begins with asking the right question.[11] When we need to find evidence for an individual patient—such as a patient with CAP—the task is relatively straightforward. A patient has a clinical condition, some diagnostic or therapeutic approach is not clear, and the evidence is reviewed and appraised to guide the clinical decision making. (Of course, skills in finding and appraising evidence must be part of the repertoire.) Asking the right question for system-level improvement is sometimes a little bit different.

Types of Questions

Questions to find evidence can be categorized in several ways. A question might look for a definitive answer (for example, "What are the most common causes of hyponatremia in a patient with liver disease?"). Alternatively, a question might inquire about information that is less definitive (for example, "Why did this patient with liver disease develop ascites now?"). In the former case, the answer will be a specific list of the most common causes of hyponatremia in patients with liver disease. In the latter, the answer will provide a range of options, but the clinician(s) can only surmise *why* this occurred at this time. Similarly, questions for finding evidence can be specific knowledge-based questions, such as "What are the diagnostic criteria for diastolic heart failure?" These types of questions are "background questions" and are most commonly asked when an individual does not have a lot of clinical experience (*see* Figure 2-3 on page 20). Background questions are used to fill the gaps in one's knowledge base.[11]

FIGURE 2-3. *Clinical Experience Versus the Number of Background Questions and Foreground Questions**

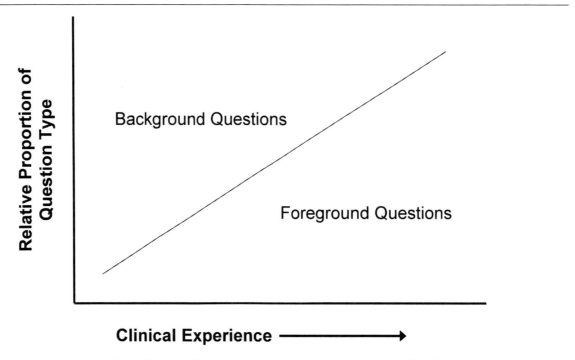

*As clinical experience increases, the number of background questions about a topic decreases and the number of foreground questions increases. Experience is a necessary component to asking foreground questions.

The PICO method. As experience increases, the types of questions that one asks change accordingly. Foreground questions, which are patient centered,[11] begin to develop. The PICO (which stands for patient, intervention, comparison, outcome) method can help ensure that a question is patient centered and specific:

- **Patient:** Ask a question that has a definite focus for a specific patient. For example, "In this 82-year-old man with severe diastolic dysfunction, . . ."
- **Intervention:** Describe the diagnostic test, therapy, or prognostic factor that we need to know more about, such as "angiotensin-converting enzyme (ACE) inhibitor medicine for diastolic dysfunction."
- **Comparison:** Determine what standard to compare to either the patient or the intervention, such as "How do ACE inhibitors compare to angiotensin II receptor blockers (ARBs)?"
- **Outcome:** Specify the clinical or diagnostic outcome to evaluate, such as "symptom relief in patients with diastolic dysfunction."[11]

Putting this all together, we create a comprehensive foreground of clinical questions that we can use to find evidence:

In an 82-year-old man with severe cardiac diastolic dysfunction, what is the efficacy of symptom reduction when using an ARB versus an ACE inhibitor?

The background question about diagnostic criteria for diastolic dysfunction seeks a specific answer, while the foreground question delves more deeply into relative strengths and weaknesses of certain medications. You can see that both types of questions are important and that each has a role when we're looking for evidence.

Questions to Find Evidence on Populations and Systems

Background and foreground questions can be framed to find the best evidence for populations of patients and systems. For example, one might ask a background question such as "What percentage of patients have diastolic dysfunction?" This question inquires into the epidemiology and background information regarding diastolic dysfunction for populations with congestive heart failure. It does not, however, address the epidemiology of diastolic dysfunction within a particular location or context. This would require a foreground question about a specific population of patients. Using the PICO method, we may inquire, "In our population of patients (*P*) with diastolic heart failure at Lake Pines Medical Center, what antihypertensive medications (*I* and *C*) should be recommended to decrease their symptoms?" This foreground population question localizes the evidence, focusing it on knowledge of the diagnosis and treatment of the condition in a specific population.

Filtered and Unfiltered Questions, "Right" and Best Answers

Background questions tend to be more general and knowledge based, while foreground questions probe that knowledge in order to apply it in a specific way—whether for an individual patient (an 82-year-old man with diastolic dysfunction) or for a population of patients (Lake Pines Medical Center patients with diastolic dysfunction). Foreground questions are sometimes more challenging to formulate than background questions because one needs clinical experience to formulate them. Also, answers to background questions have often been filtered (that is, assessed and compiled by others[12]) and the "right" answers are therefore easy to identify in textbooks or general review articles. It is often simple to identify a list of diagnostic features or treatment options for a particular condition, and this background information is essential before we progress to the more complex foreground questions. Answers to foreground questions may not be available in the same way. The literature may not provide a definite "right" answer, but it can be used to determine the *best* answer to guide care at that particular time. This is where the balance of the components of EBP becomes important (*see* Figure 2-1 on page 17).

As we said at the beginning of this section, forming the right question is a key first step in finding the right evidence. Having the right question involves knowledge of the situation, and this is true whether we are searching for information for an individual patient or looking for information to apply across a particular population. Getting the question right is the necessary starting point in finding the information and applying it to a specific patient care situation.

Evaluating the Strength of Evidence

Many available resources discuss the strength of evidence. In this book, we do not provide a comprehensive evaluation of research methodology or a detailed discussion of the relative strengths and weaknesses of study design and biostatistics. However, we do offer a few key points that will help you evaluate the relative strength of evidence you find.

Figure 2-4 below is a pyramid diagram that summarizes the relative strength of research evidence based on the study design or resource type.[12] The quality and strength of evidence increases from the base of the pyramid to the peak. The lower half of the pyramid contains unfiltered information, while the upper part contains reviews and syntheses that have been filtered.

Unfiltered Information

At the base of the pyramid are expert opinions, case reports, and case-controlled studies. These are usually anecdotal reports of interesting findings or a consensus

FIGURE 2-4. *Pyramid Diagram Representing the Relative Strength of Evidence of Various Forms of Information* *

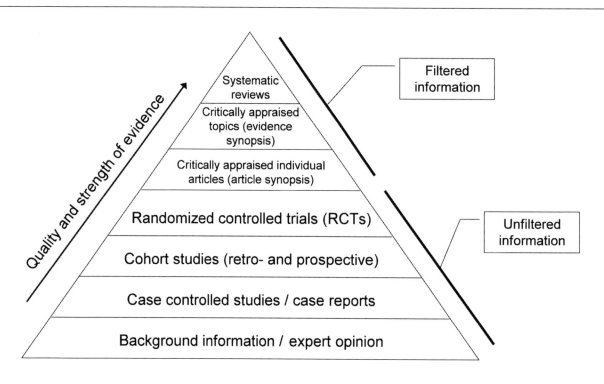

* Although the evidence at the top of the pyramid is considered to be the highest quality, it also has been assessed and compiled by others—that is, the information has been filtered.

Source: Dartmouth Medical Libraries: *Evidence-Based Medicine (EBM) Resources.* http://www.dartmouth.edu/~biomed/resources.htmld/guides.ebm_resources .shtml (accessed May 17, 2011). Reprinted with permission from Karen V. Odato, Research and Education Librarian, Dartmouth Biomedical Libraries.

statement from a panel of experts about a condition for which a higher level of evidence does not yet exist. Although these often contain detailed stories of individual cases, they are considered less strong than other types of evidence because there is no experimental design. Although rich narrative information that is particular to a case or cases might provide some guidance, it generally does not provide the strength of evidence required to make system-level changes.

Cohort studies. Further up the pyramid, but still falling within unfiltered information, are cohort studies, both retrospective and prospective. Cohort studies follow a group of individuals over a period of time. For these studies, a large amount of data is collected about each individual, and the analysis takes into account the time of the observation period—which may be many years—and the complex interactions between the factors collected. Many health services research projects that employ analysis of large databases are either prospective or retrospective cohort analyses.

RCTs. Randomized controlled trials (RCTs) comprise the final level of unfiltered information. These are usually held as the gold standard for building scientific knowledge. RCTs are considered strong evidence because they control for as many factors as possible, both in the design and in the statistical analysis of these projects. Randomization has the added benefit of controlling for unknown as well as known factors that might influence the outcome. The control group in an RCT provides a comparison to identify whether the changes in the intervention group are due to the intervention or due to an underlying characteristic of the group as a whole. Meta-analysis (not pictured in Figure 2-4) combines data from many studies in an effort to pool information and arrive at a conclusion.

Filtered Information

Above RCTs on the pyramid are sources of filtered information. These sources appraise the evidence and usually offer recommendations for practice. They may be summaries and evaluations of individual journal articles (article synopses) or syntheses of evidence from many sources (evidence syntheses). Filtered information is often convenient because someone else has gone through it and created a summary of the main findings.

Evidence syntheses. An evidence synthesis can include evidence from a range of studies on the topic, including RCTs, cohort studies, and expert opinions. The National Guideline Clearinghouse accessed by the medical, nursing, and pharmacy students in the opening vignette is an example of an evidence synthesis, where the guidelines vary in quality from those based on expert opinions to those based on higher-quality research evidence.

Systematic reviews. At the top of the pyramid are systematic reviews, such as the Cochrane Database of Systematic Reviews. The Cochrane Collaboration is an international not-for-profit organization that was established in 1993 to prepare, update, and promote the accessibility of systematic reviews of the health care literature.

The Cochrane Library
http://www.cochrane.org

To date, there are more than 4,600 reviews published online in *The Cochrane Library*. (For more information, visit http://www.cochrane.org.) Systematic reviews are generated by experts who complete structured comprehensive literature reviews, evaluate the literature, and present summaries of the findings.

Consider the perspective of filtered information. When researching filtered information, it is important to understand the perspective of the authors and the sponsoring agency. For example, an evidence synopsis about CAP sponsored by an organization of infectious disease professionals will likely contain a focus different from that of a similar review sponsored by a home care organization. One of them may focus on the microbiology and pharmacology for treating pneumonia, while the other may focus on nonpharmacologic interventions to help patients recuperate at home. Both foci are valid and important, but understanding the perspective from which a review is written will help in interpreting the information.

Level of Evidence

Identifying the level of evidence is an important step when reviewing the information. The level of evidence is a by-product of the rigor of the research design. Making generalizations from case study–level data is not wise. Also, just because an article is written as a review does not mean that it contains valid conclusions or is the final word on a topic. An extensive review of all levels of evidence for a particular condition (such as CAP) is not always needed. The goal is to find the best available evidence. For example, if a well-done, recent systematic review or meta-analysis is available that directly answers the clinical question at hand, then the search can end. If the systematic review is well done but not recent, we would want to look for any RCTs done since it was published to see if there is any new evidence. If a systematic review is not available at all, then we'd look for RCTs (the study type that provides the highest-quality evidence for therapy). If we then find relevant RCTs, we could appraise them and use their evidence. If there are no RCTs, then we would look for case-controlled studies, case series, or a case study. We would search for the highest quality of evidence available to answer our particular question. The trick is finding it.

Choosing the Right Resource Based on the Question

Many electronic resources are available and are continually updated and improved. The sheer number of resources can be overwhelming, and often we become familiar and comfortable with one or two of the most common resources. While the specific resources may change over time, it is useful to be familiar with different search interfaces. Each interface has a role in finding evidence.

Table 2-1 (*see* pages 25–26), originally developed at the Dartmouth Biomedical Libraries in Hanover, New Hampshire, is a helpful quick guide for finding evidence-based answers to clinical questions. The resources available from your local biomedical library may be similar, and resources will likely evolve over time.[13]

TABLE 2-1.
Resources for Finding Answers to Clinical Questions

What Is Needed	Examples	Resources to Consider
An overview of a particular disease, condition (background information)	What's the difference between depression and bipolar disorder? I have a new patient with sickle cell anemia; I need an overview of this condition.	Textbooks (print or online) UpToDate eMedicine
Drug information	What is the pediatric dosage of erythromycin for strep throat? What drugs have been approved by the FDA for the treatment of Alzheimer's?	Clinical Pharmacology Online Epocrates Online Drug Facts and Comparisons (print) or USP-DI MEDLINE for more specific information Embase (Scopus) ClinicalTrials.gov (registry and results database of federally and privately funded clinical trials)
A synthesis of best-practice recommendations for disease management (critically appraised topics)	What's the latest on the management of panic disorder? What's the best method of pain control in children?	Cochrane Database Clinical evidence MEDLINE (Clinical Queries—Systematic Reviews category) National Guideline Clearinghouse MEDLINE (limit to "Practice Guidelines" publication type) TRIP (simultaneously searches multiple evidence-based resources)
An answer to a narrow question that isn't addressed in the synthesis resources (critically appraised articles and unfiltered information)	In a 70-year-old woman with primary insomnia and a previous adverse reaction to hypnotics, can cognitive behavior therapy improve sleep quality and duration? In a toddler with croup, does dexamethasone (or another glucocorticoid) reduce symptoms better than standard supportive care?	MEDLINE (Clinical Queries—Clinical Study Category) ACP Journal Club *BMJ* updates TRIP ClinicalTrials.gov Embase (Scopus)
Evidence-based information about alternative therapies	Is melatonin safe and effective for treating insomnia? Does music therapy help surgical patients heal faster?	MEDLINE (limit to "Complementary Medicine" subset and "RCT" publication type) Alternative and complementary medicine resources [for example, the Allied and Complementary Medicine Database (AMED)] TRIP Embase (Scopus)

(continued)

TABLE 2-1.

Resources for Finding Answers to Clinical Questions *(continued)*

Cutting-edge information that isn't yet published in the journal literature (not necessarily evidence based)	My patient heard about a new drug on the news last night. The drug is so new that it's not in CPO or MEDLINE. Where can I find more information about it?	News resources (LexisNexis) Web resources (Google; Google Scholar) ClinicalTrials.gov
Information to share with patients	Where can I find some nutrition information for a patient who has been newly diagnosed with diabetes?	MEDLINEPlus.gov Informed Health online Other consumer health resources

Source: Biomedical Libraries Web Group: *Finding Evidence-Based Answers to Clinical Questions—Quickly and Effectively.* http://www.dartmouth.edu/~biomed/resources.htmld/guides/FindingGoodAnswers.pdf (accessed Jul. 13, 2011). Adapted with permission from Dartmouth Biomedical Libraries.

TRIP Database

http://www.tripdatabase.com

For example, when we need an overview of a particular condition (background question), print or online textbooks or summary sites are very helpful; however, summary sites will likely not contain enough detailed information if the question has a narrow focus or if we need information about a topic that was published in the past several months. One resource, Turning Research into Practice (TRIP), at http://www.tripdatabase.com, is freely available and searches many databases at once. The TRIP Database casts a wide net through evidence-based sources of systematic reviews, practice guidelines, and critically appraised topics and articles, as well as MEDLINE's Clinical Queries, medical image databases, e-textbooks, and patient information leaflets. If the question encompasses a unique aspect, such as alternative therapies, or if we want to find cutting-edge information, then resources such as MEDLINE with "complementary medicine" limits for indexed journal articles or LexisNexis for news resources would provide the best options.

This list is not a comprehensive compendium of every available database or search engine, but it is a reasonable starting point for finding evidence based on the need. Each of the resources listed here has strengths and limitations. Searching them on your own is a practical place to start. When you need very detailed information, however, connecting with a reference librarian is the most sensible option.

Working with a Reference Librarian

Not long ago—as recently as the late 1990s—databases for finding evidence were not user friendly. The Internet was still in its infancy, and few institutions had high-speed Internet connections. Most libraries used a telnet connection over telephone lines that were quite slow, even for material without graphics. The interface with these tools was not a simple Web browser; rather, it required a case-sensitive and punctuation-sensitive string of characters. Reference librarians used cryptic strings of characters to retrieve evidence for clinicians and researchers. Those librarians—with master's degrees and usually on staff at biomedical libraries affiliated with medical schools—were expert mediators for literature searches.

With the continued development of evidence search engines such as MEDLINE via Ovid or PubMed or even Google Scholar, we have entered an era of independent end-user searchers. These interfaces appear simple. Many offer onscreen help and instructions, and most provide check boxes for narrowing the search criteria. The apparent simplicity in these interfaces sometimes comes at the expense of a careful, detailed search for the strongest and most reliable evidence on a topic. For a variety of reasons, ranging from a do-it-yourself mentality to embarrassment at asking for help to simply not knowing about the expertise of librarians, most clinicians and researchers no longer enlist the help of a reference librarian.

Levels of Literature Searches

Whether you need to use a reference librarian may depend on the level of your literature search. There are three broad levels of literature searches:

- **Level 1—Rapid searches:** The goal of these searches is to be quick. A rapid search is a broad stroke to capture as many resources as possible. These searches are not limited by many—if any—modifiers. Google Scholar currently operates in this fashion, identifying the range of resources available for a topic. The number of hits with this type of search is often quite large.
- **Level 2—Careful searches:** Careful searches often start by planning the search strategy. The searcher pays close attention to the literature types and resources that may be searched (for example, specific journals, newspaper articles, and online resources). You may start with Google Scholar but will likely need to move to a PubMed or Ovid interface in order to limit your search appropriately. After a set of resources is found, you can further manipulate them by limiting the set. A reference librarian is a tremendous asset for these searches.
- **Level 3—Expert searches:** Expert searches truly demand the assistance of a reference librarian. This type of search is necessary when you need to find clinical information for a very specific question or for a rare clinical condition. Perhaps you plan on publishing a systematic review or a meta-analysis. In this case, the search will be scrutinized, and expert assistance will make the process stronger.

Reference librarians are an often-untapped source of guidance for improvement work. They are highly trained specialists who can find what you need faster and better than you can on your own. Sometimes they can even help you formulate questions. Just as improvement work on the front lines requires input from all health professionals (*see* Chapter 3), expert help can enhance the search for the best evidence for improvement.

Summary

Because improving patient care involves closing the gap between the right care and current local performance, finding the right evidence is an important first step in improvement work. Evidence comes in many forms, and we should always search for the strongest evidence available. EBP precepts and tools need to be applied in health care systems and not just on a patient-by-patient basis. In short, improving care for patients requires that the best evidence be reliably applied to the right patients at the right time.

References

1. Oxman A.D., Sackett D.L., Guyatt G.H.: Users' guides to the medical literature: I. How to get started. *JAMA* 270:2093–2095, Nov. 3, 1993.

2. Guyatt G.H., Sackett D.L., Cook D.J.: Users' guides to the medical literature: II. How to use an article about therapy or prevention. A. Are the results of the study valid? *JAMA* 270:2598–2601, Dec. 1, 1993.

3. Guyatt G.H., Sackett D.L., Cook D.J.: Users' guides to the medical literature: II. How to use an article about therapy or prevention. B. What were the results and will they help me in caring for my patients? *JAMA* 271:59–63, Jan. 5, 1994.

4. Jaeschke R., Guyatt G.H., Sackett D.L.: Users' guides to the medical literature: III. How to use an article about a diagnostic test. A. Are the results of the study valid? *JAMA* 271:389–391, Feb. 2, 1994.

5. Jaeschke R., Guyatt G.H., Sackett D.L.: Users' guides to the medical literature: III. How to use an article about a diagnostic test. B. What are the results and will they help me in caring for my patients? *JAMA* 271:703–707, Mar. 2, 1994.

6. Cullen L., et al.: Sigma Theta Tau international position statement on evidence-based practice February 2007 summary. *Worldviews Evid Based Nurs* 5:57–59, Jun. 6, 2008.

7. Goode, C.J., et al.: The Colorado Patient-Centered Interprofessional Evidence-Based Practice Model: A framework for transformation. *Worldviews Evid Based Nurs* 8:96–105, Dec. 6, 2010.

8. Lewis S.: Toward a general theory of indifference to research-based evidence. *J Health Serv Res Policy* 12:166–172, Jul. 1, 2007.

9. Scott I.A.: The evolving science of translating research evidence into clinical practice. *ACP J Club* 146:A8–A11, May–Jun. 2007.

10. Batalden P.B., Davidoff F.: What is "quality improvement" and how can it transform healthcare? *Qual Saf Health Care* 16:2–3, Feb. 2007.

11. Bauman N.: *How to Research the Medical Literature: Framing Specific Foreground and Background Questions in an Evidence-Based Way.* Nov. 1, 2001. http://www.nasw.org/users/nbauman/habrown.htm (accessed May 17, 2011).

12. Dartmouth Medical Libraries: *Evidence-Based Medicine (EBM) Resources.* http://www.dartmouth.edu/~biomed/resources.htmld/guides.ebm_resources.shtml (accessed May 17, 2011).

13. Biomedical Libraries Web Group: *Finding Evidence-Based Answers to Clinical Questions—Quickly and Effectively.* http://www.dartmouth.edu/~biomed/resources.htmld/guides/FindingGoodAnswers.pdf (accessed Jul. 13, 2011).

CHAPTER 3

Working in Interprofessional Teams for the Improvement of Patient Care

OBJECTIVES

After reading this chapter, you will be able to do the following:

1. Identify the criteria for effective teamwork and the outcomes of a successful team.
2. Recognize the characteristics of the professionals who work together to provide safe and effective care to patients.
3. Describe factors that influence team functioning and how to assess them.
4. Choose members to be part of an interprofessional health care improvement team.

Phong Nguyen, an attending physician, walks to the inpatient medicine unit to meet with Carlos Velasquez, the unit nurse manager. Over the past several weeks, the inpatient team has been working on increasing the number of patients receiving the influenza vaccine. Phong and Carlos, each with a background in improvement and systems, have been leading the team through a small project to demonstrate that it is possible to improve care as part of the usual day-to-day work in an inpatient medicine unit. In addition to Phong and Carlos, the team includes a clinical pharmacist, a staff nurse, a resident, an intern, a medical student, and a nursing student. The first several weeks of this project have gone very well. The team started with a flu vaccine rate of about 40%, improved to over 80% within three weeks, and peaked at a 100% vaccination rate in the fourth week (see Figure 3-1 on page 30). The team members have been extremely enthusiastic about this process because it has been focused, measurable, and doable within the four-week time frame that the learners spend in the unit.

When the team members gather, they turn their attention to the whiteboard containing the information about their flu vaccine improvement project. The whiteboard displays the project's aim at the top, a small graph of the outcomes of the work, and a list of the changes the team members have tried (see Figure 3-2 on page 31). As is typical for improvement efforts, the team members started by looking for technological fixes and by professing increased vigilance for flu vaccines. It wasn't until they made flu vaccines a routine part of their assessment and plan for each patient that the rate of vaccination increased. Last week the team decided that the best way to integrate flu vaccines into the system of care was to enable nurses to evaluate the need for a vaccine and to administer it without an order from the physician (that is, they needed a standing order for flu vaccine). The pharmacist on the team was able to develop a process to streamline vaccine dispensing so that this additional duty would not be burdensome for already busy nurses.

The team is pleased with its success and recognizes that it is due in part to the commitment to including all *members of the care team in the improvement efforts.*

Teams in the Health Care Setting

Whether as part of a Little League baseball team, the high school drama club, or a care team on a medicine ward, almost everyone has experience working in teams. We are inundated with the terms *team* and *teamwork* in the media, in sports, and in management books. Sometimes team members are expected to complete every task together, but teams are complex, and not all tasks require a team approach.[1] In addition, a team is not just a group of individuals assembled; teams require proper formation and management.

FIGURE 3-1. *Whiteboard Used in Team Room to Track the Aim and Data of an Improvement Project*

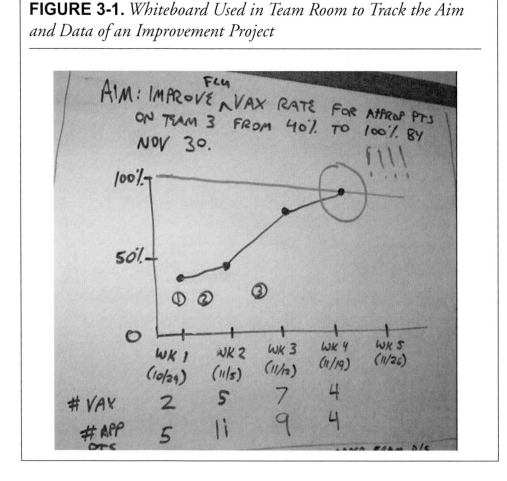

FIGURE 3-2. *List of Changes Tried over the Weeks of the Flu Vaccine Improvement Project*

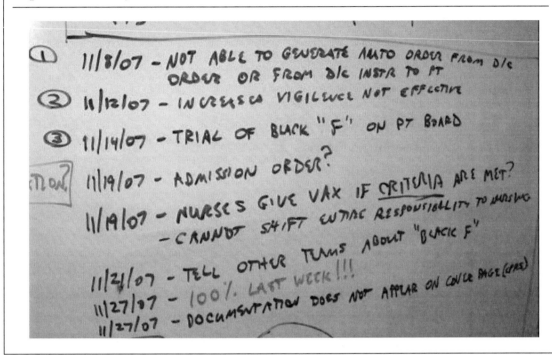

While most of us spend a good deal of time in teams (in both our professional and personal lives), we are typically not taught how to form or manage them. This chapter, serving as a basic overview of teams for improving health care, includes the following information:

- A basic taxonomy of types of teams
- The benefits of the team approach
- Skills that teams need in order to be successful
- Guidance on factors that influence team functioning
- Guidance on how to assess teams
- Descriptions of some of the professions that come together to provide patient care and the role that they play in improving care

Focus and Commitment

One definition for *team* is "a group of people working together to achieve a common purpose for which they hold themselves mutually accountable."[2(pp.1–2)] Teams are useful for completing complex tasks and developing insights into a system. A productive team must have a clearly defined goal to understand *what* it is trying to accomplish and *why*. Purpose gives the team direction and offers a sense of value and commitment. This includes understanding to whom the team reports and how the team measures the success of its work. Although teams can be effective at working across disciplines and departments, a team will be more effective if it can maintain its focus and work within its locus of control.

One definition for team is "a group of people working together to achieve a common purpose for which they hold themselves mutually accountable."

Teams require commitment from individuals and from the organization to get work done, so it is important to carefully choose the times when and places where teams are needed. For example, in the opening vignette, the goal of the inpatient medicine team is to evaluate, make diagnoses, and direct and administer therapies for patients as well as to teach young health care professionals. This team is a constant presence on the inpatient service and is an example of a *work team*.

Work Teams

Work teams tend to be long-standing fixtures that bear responsibility for completing tasks in a particular setting. For example, the opening vignette's inpatient medicine team was assembled to provide care for patients and training for the learners, and it includes members with different levels of experience and members of different professions. Even though each has a different level of experience and different training, they come together to provide care to the patients on the inpatient medical service. As another example, a neonatal intensive care unit (ICU) work team might include the attending neonatologist, a fellow, a pediatric resident, a medical student, a nurse, a dietitian, a pharmacist, a social worker, and a case manager. Often the patient's family is also included on this type of work team. Clinical work teams are stable and predictable groups in many settings.

Project Teams

In contrast to work teams, which tend to focus on a particular setting, *project teams* focus on specific problems. Quality improvement work often occurs in project teams. In the opening vignette, the work team of the medicine unit had also formed into a project team to increase the rate of influenza vaccination.

Criteria for forming a project team. When the following four criteria exist in a challenging situation, forming a project team will likely be more effective than individual efforts[3]:
1. The task is complex, and no one person has all the knowledge or skills needed to solve the task.
2. Creativity is required.
3. The testing of changes will require commitment and cooperation across units or departments.
4. The task being examined is cross-functional and involves several professions.

As the clinical team in our example discovered, even something as seemingly straightforward as reliably providing influenza vaccines can become complex very quickly. No one person (or profession) has cornered the market on the knowledge and skills needed to improve the system. Involving many perspectives in a project team allows creativity to flourish, and the group is more likely to come up with creative ideas. The team realized that although the physician orders the vaccine, the pharmacist dispenses it and the nurse administers it. When the team decided to recommend a standing order, it made this recommendation with input from all health professionals involved in the unit. The team was successful because it recommended changes with full knowledge of the process of care—knowledge it had because of the interprofessional nature of the team.

Improvement Teams

Properly formed teams rely on the knowledge, skills, and experience of a wide range of people to solve problems. The dynamic interaction of the individuals helps them make good decisions and find effective solutions. But what are the components of an effective improvement team?

An improvement team should include an individual with enough authority in the organization to institute a change. This person is the team's system leader; he or she understands the implications of the changes and can interact with other system leaders.[3] In our example, Phong and Carlos would have the responsibilities for system leadership. An improvement team also needs team members with technical expertise who understand the day-to-day workings of the system. In our example, the intern who writes orders, the pharmacist who knows about the dispensing of vaccines, and the staff nurses who administer vaccines on the inpatient unit bring this perspective. These individuals understand how the systems operate and what an effective intervention strategy might include. An improvement project team also requires an individual for day-to-day leadership—someone who is part of the process on a daily basis. The resident plays this role with the guidance of Carlos, the nurse manager. Another important addition to the team is an executive sponsor. This is an individual in a top management position with whom the team leader(s) has open communication. The executive sponsor is generally in a position to provide resources or remove barriers that the team may experience.

> **Improvement Team**
> *An improvement team should include the following members:*
> - *System leader*
> - *Team members with technical expertise*
> - *Day-to-day leader(s)*
> - *Executive sponsor*

Currently, most health care improvement teams are project teams. While we know these teams can be effective, there is an inherent weakness to this approach: "Project work" remains outside the scope of usual daily tasks and often is considered to be additional work. The influenza vaccine team tried to incorporate improvement into its daily routine but realized that its efforts were limited because of the composition of the team. Improvement activities in health care will remain project team activities until work teams are redesigned. Neonatal ICUs and outpatient interprofessional spine centers have demonstrated that this transformation is possible.[4,5] As health care improvement becomes part and parcel of providing care, improvement activities will become a core function of clinical work teams.

Interprofessional Teams for Improvement

Teams and teamwork form the backbone of quality improvement work, and an interprofessional composition makes a team come to life. While some may use the terms *interdisciplinary* or even *multidisciplinary*, we favor the term *interprofessional*. The term *interdisciplinary* may be confusing because it can also mean cooperation between disciplines in a single field such as medicine; for example, pediatrics, surgery, and anesthesia are all disciplines within the field of medicine. Furthermore, the prefix *multi-* suggests that members can work independently toward a common goal, but the prefix *inter-* points to a collaborative effort.[6] Patients benefit from receiving care from a team of health professionals with expertise specific to their individual problems. With assistance from the patient as well as paraprofessionals, an interprofessional team provides a depth of knowledge and skills that surpasses the expertise of any one person.

Becoming Familiar with Health Care Professional Characteristics

Because most current professional education involves students from the same profession working together to master a specific body of knowledge and skills, health professions students often enter clinical care with little interprofessional knowledge or experience. They arrive in a clinic or on a hospital unit and must interact with physicians, nurses, pharmacists, and health administrators, even though they have never been taught how those interactions can occur for the benefit of patients. Many students lack even a basic understanding of the training and background of other health professionals.

Table 3-1 on pages 35–36 provides a summary of key characteristics of physicians, nurses, pharmacists, and health care administrators. Other health care professionals, such as physician assistants, advance practice nurses, dietitians, and physical therapists, play a significant role in performance improvement as well. This table, which was prepared with assistance from educational leaders in each of the professions it highlights, summarizes the key values, educational pathways, and important historical facts related to these professions. Note the similarities across the rows. For example, the key values of each profession focus on improving care for patients. This common focus is the tie that binds all health care professions. When care providers are frustrated by processes or poor outcomes, refocusing on patients and their families is an effective way to bring health care professionals together. Also, the educational pathway for each profession requires didactic classroom learning coupled with experiential learning. This experiential learning is an opportunity to apply the knowledge and skills learned in the classroom to real-world scenarios; however, this experience often occurs without the presence of other health professionals or students.

The Need for Interprofessional Education

Because everyone works together for patients after training is completed, some of the clinical training for all the professions should include interprofessional experiences. In fact, the World Health Organization (WHO) reports that "there is now sufficient evidence to indicate that interprofessional education enables effective collaborative practice which in turn optimizes health-services, strengthens health systems and improves health outcomes."[7(p.18)] The WHO model for interprofessional education is presented in Figure 3-3 on page 37.

National efforts to reinforce these recommendations also exist. The Canadian Interprofessional Health Collaborative was founded in 2006 to integrate projects

---

Because most current professional education involves students from the same profession working together to master a specific body of knowledge and skills, health professions students often enter clinical care with little interprofessional knowledge or experience.

The World Health Organization (WHO) reports that "there is now sufficient evidence to indicate that interprofessional education enables effective collaborative practice which in turn optimizes health-services, strengthens health systems and improves health outcomes."

TABLE 3-1.
Key Characteristics of Health Care Professionals

	Physician*	Nurse†	Pharmacist‡	Health Care Administrator
Key Values of the Profession	• Competence • Honesty with patients • Patient confidentiality • Appropriate relationships with patients • Improved quality of care • Improved access to care • Just distribution of finite resources • Scientific knowledge • Maintenance of trust through management of conflicts of interest	• Competence • Integrity • Compassion and respect for the inherent dignity of all patients • Primacy of commitment to the patient, whether an individual, a family, or the community • Effective collaboration with other team members to achieve health goals of patients • Protection of the health, safety, and rights of patients • Maintenance of competence, improved work environments, and improved quality of care	• Welfare of humanity and relief of suffering • Application of knowledge, experience, and skills to ensure optimal outcomes for patients • Respect for and protection of all personal and health information • Obligation to improve professional knowledge and competence • Highest principles of moral, ethical, and legal conduct • Changes that improve patient care • Utilization of knowledge, skills, experiences, and values to educate and train the next generation of pharmacists	• Competence • Teamwork • Fiduciary duty • Efficiency and effectiveness • High ethical standards • Organizational change • Relationships with all stakeholder groups • Leadership
Educational Pathway	• Four-year undergraduate degree • Four years of medical school • Postgraduate residency training in a specialty (three to eight years)	• Two to four years of undergraduate coursework to become eligible for basic R.N. licensure exam (A.D.N. or B.S.N. degree) • Two to three years graduate education (M.S.N. or D.N.P.) to become eligible for certification as advanced practice nurse (C.R.N.A., C.N.M., N.P., C.N.L., or C.N.S.)	• Two to four years of undergraduate coursework • Four years of pharmacy school • Voluntary postgraduate residency training for one to two years	• B.S. in health care administration for entry-level positions • Masters of health administration (M.H.A. or equivalent) for middle and executive management • One-year postgraduate fellowship desirable but not required

(continued)

TABLE 3-1.

Key Characteristics of Health Care Professionals *(continued)*

Important Historical Facts	• The first medical school in the United States was founded in 1765. • Most medical schools today still follow the curriculum (two years in the classroom and two years of clerkship) recommended by Abraham Flexner in 1912.	• Florence Nightingale pioneered nursing schools in 1860 when she opened the Nightingale Training School for Nurses. • In the United States, the first autonomous (non-hospital-service-based) nursing school opened in 1923 as the Yale School of Nursing. • Nurses comprise the largest group of health care workers in the United States.	• The first pharmacy school in the United States was founded in 1821. • Movement to a doctoral level of training began in 1960 and was mandated in 2000.	• Formal health administration education started at the University of Chicago in 1934 and at Northwestern University in 1943. • The Association of University Programs in Health Administration (AUPHA) brings together more than 140 certified undergraduate and accredited graduate health care management programs from across North America.

Note: Other health care professionals, such as physician assistants, advance practice nurses, dietitians, and physical therapists, play a significant role in performance improvement as well.

* The key values for the physician are modified from the American Board of Internal Medicine (ABIM) recommendations regarding professionalism.
† The key values for the nurse are modified from the American Nurses Association Code of Ethics.
‡ The key values for the pharmacist are modified from "The Oath of the Pharmacist," updated and approved by the American Association of Colleges of Pharmacy House of Delegates in July 2007.

carried out through the Interprofessional Education for Collaborative, Patient-Centred Practice. In 2011 in the United States, the Interprofessional Education Collaborative (IPEC) released competencies to advance collaborative practice. The four competency domains are values/ethics for interprofessional practice, roles/responsibilities, interprofessional communication, and teams and teamwork. The general competency statement for teams and teamwork is to "apply relationship-building values and the principles of team dynamics to perform effectively in different team roles to plan and deliver patient-/population-centered care that is safe, timely, efficient, effective, and equitable."[8(p.25)] Specific competencies for teams and teamwork are listed in Table 3-2 on page 38.

Furthermore, the Institute of Medicine (IOM) makes this recommendation: "All health professionals should be educated to deliver patient-centered care as members of an interdisciplinary team, emphasizing evidence-based practice, quality improvement approaches, and informatics."[9] The recommendations identified by the IOM were further defined as competencies and delineated through the Quality and Safety Education for Nurses (QSEN) initiative.[10] Even though the effort targeted nursing education in the United States, perusal of the knowledge, skill, and attitude elements comprising the competency for teamwork and collaboration provide appropriate guidance in competency development for all health professions students. These can be conveniently found on the QSEN Web site, at http://www.qsen.org.

QSEN

http://www.qsen.org

Enhancing Team Functioning

As noted previously, effective teamwork is not a concept that has been historically included in health professions curriculum. Teams can't be expected to function well without some guidance on *how* to function well.

Factors That Influence Team Functioning

Key factors that influence team functioning include communication style and authority gradients. Collaborative and assertive communication has been demonstrated to have a positive effect on patient outcomes.[11] Indeed, focusing on communicating the needs of patients is also useful in dealing with authority gradients. Authority gradients occur when a health professional (or student) is hesitant to share pertinent information with a more senior colleague or with someone who has more perceived (or actual) power in the organizational structure.

Authority gradients occur when a health professional (or student) is hesitant to share pertinent information with a more senior colleague or with someone who has more perceived (or actual) power in the organizational structure.

Structured communication methods. Following are two examples of effective structured communication methods that may help team functioning:

1. **Situation–Background–Assessment–Recommendation (SBAR)**[12]:
   This method is a structured communication approach that assists health

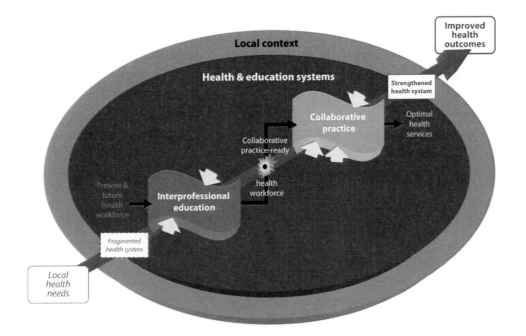

FIGURE 3-3. *The World Health Organization Model for Interprofessional Education*

Source: Health Professions Networks, Nursing & Midwifery, Human Resources for Health: *Framework for Action on Interprofessional Education & Collaborative Practice*. Geneva: World Health Organization, 2010. http://whqlibdoc.who.int/hq/2010/WHO_HRH_HPN_10.3_eng.pdf (accessed May 19, 2011). Reprinted with permission.

professionals in communicating relevant patient information in a concise and focused approach. *Situation* is a one-sentence description of what is going on. *Background* provides clinical or contextual details. *Assessment* describes what the communicator thinks is going on. Finally, the specific approach to solve the problem or need is suggested as a *recommendation*.

2. **The Three W's**[13]: Used in crew resource management training in the Veterans Health Administration system, this technique's format involves the statements "What I see . . ." "What I am concerned about . . ." and "What I want."

Gauging the Effectiveness of Interprofessional Teamwork

Once teams are formed, it is important to assess their effectiveness. The Agency for Healthcare Research and Quality (AHRQ) offers two tools through its TeamSTEPPS® (Strategies and Tools to Enhance Performance and Patient Safety) program, which teaches leadership, communication, mutual support, and situation monitoring.[14] One tool assesses individual *attitudes* toward teamwork (capturing how an individual

---

TABLE 3-2.
Specific Team and Teamwork Competencies

1. Describe the process of team development and the roles and practices of effective teams.

2. Develop consensus on the ethical principles to guide all aspects of patient care and teamwork.

3. Engage other health professionals—appropriate to the specific care situation—in shared patient-centered problem solving.

4. Integrate the knowledge and experience of other professions—appropriate to the specific care situation—to inform care decisions while respecting patient and community values and priorities/preferences for care.

5. Apply leadership practices that support collaborative practice and team effectiveness.

6. Engage self and others to constructively manage disagreements about values, roles, goals, and actions that arise among health care professionals and with patients and families.

7. Share accountability with other professions, patients, and communities for outcomes relevant to prevention and health care.

8. Reflect on individual and team performance for the improvement of both.

9. Use process improvement strategies to increase the effectiveness of interprofessional teamwork and team-based care.

10. Use available evidence to inform effective teamwork and team-based practices.

11. Perform effectively on teams and in different team roles in a variety of settings.

Source: Interprofessional Education Collaborative Expert Panel: *Core Competencies for Interprofessional Collaborative Practice: Report of an Expert Panel.* Washington, DC: Interprofessional Education Collaborative, 2011.

approaches team-related issues), while the other assesses individual *perceptions* of group-level teamwork (measuring how an individual sees the current state of teamwork in the particular setting). Both tools contribute to a true picture of how a team is functioning, as not all members of a team have similar perceptions of teamwork.[15] The University of Colorado School of Medicine offers yet another way to gauge the effectiveness of teamwork. Its first-year medical students use the tool in Figure 3-4 on page 40 to rate the hospital teams they shadow. By observing teams and reflecting on their observations, the students increase their awareness of the factors that contribute to team success.

Interaction of Health Professionals in Specific Clinical Situations

Clearly, the complexity of the health care environment requires the expertise of a variety of health professionals. The examples in Table 3-3 on page 41 show a range of clinical scenarios and when each of the professions takes the lead in providing care. While the physician certainly has a role in each of these cases, his or her knowledge and skills will play the main role in the case of a patient with major trauma from a motor vehicle accident. However, the physician will have more of a supporting role in the case of a patient receiving hospice care at home or a patient with stable atrial fibrillation. Similarly, a nurse who provides home care for a patient receiving hospice care is the primary caregiver for that patient. The pharmacist plays an important role in helping to determine dosages and in dispensing medications for a home hospice patient. In fact, many health systems have pharmacist-run warfarin clinics to maintain safe anticoagulation for patients at risk of thromboembolism. A health care administrator is usually in the background of acute and chronic clinical care scenarios, although there are times when he or she will step to the forefront. With a patient who may have difficulty accessing care because of health insurance issues, the administrator is the person who works with the patient and family to access care through the system.

Interaction of Health Professionals in Improvement Activities

Beyond just the clinical scenarios, you can also consider how improvement activities might be led by different health care professionals. For example, if a group were working on improving the outcomes from coronary artery bypass graft surgery, a cardiothoracic surgeon might lead the improvement team. A team focusing on patient falls on the medicine wards might best be led by a nurse leader who understands the local system and can advocate for interventions to reduce falls. A team working on reducing medication errors might be led by a pharmacist. Finally, patient flow problems such as discharge planning problems could be led by a health care administrator who understands the many levels of the discharge system and how the different clinicians come together at that point in time. While these examples demonstrate who might be a reasonable leader depending on the focus of improvement, each improvement team would represent an interprofessional effort involving individuals from these and other health care professions.

FIGURE 3-4. *University of Colorado School of Medicine Clinical Interlude Hospital Team Scoring*

Team Demographics:

Team Specialty (please circle):   Anesthesia   Family Medicine   Internal Medicine   Neurology
OB/GYN   Pediatrics   Psychiatry   Surgery

Subspecialty (circle if applicable):   Cardiothoracic   Critical Care   ENT   Heme/Onc   Neurosurgery   Oncology
Orthopedics   Transplant   Urology   Vascular   Other:_____

Hospital Team Environment (please circle):   Ward/Hospital Floor   ICU/CCU   OR   Other:_____

List Team Members by Role and Number (e.g., 4 attendings, 3 RNs, 2 RTs, patient, etc.):
___Attendings   ___Fellows   ___Residents   ___Students   ___PAs   ___NPs   ___RNs   ___PTs   ___OTs   ___RTs
___PharmDs   ___Nutritionists   ___Case Managers   ___Social Workers   ___Chaplains   ___Patient   ___Family Members
___ Others:_____

Who would have been helpful on this team that is not currently a member of the team?   _____
_____
_____

Please score your hospital team based upon observations, chart reviews, and interviews by rating the following items (please circle):

Hospital Team Scoring	Always	Usually	Sometimes	Rarely	Never	Unable to Assess
Team members know the roles/responsibilities of each person on the team and understand how he or she contributes to the team's functioning.	5	4	3	2	1	U/A
Team members have roles/responsibilities that are based on their skill sets/abilities.	5	4	3	2	1	U/A
Team members are willing to be flexible in their roles/ responsibilities for the good of the team.	5	4	3	2	1	U/A
Team members share common goals.	5	4	3	2	1	U/A
Team members communicate effectively: They speak clearly and directly, are succinct, listen actively, and ask for feedback.	5	4	3	2	1	U/A
Team members regularly encourage everyone to participate.	5	4	3	2	1	U/A
Team members check for agreement.	5	4	3	2	1	U/A
Team members openly admit oversights and shortcomings.	5	4	3	2	1	U/A
Team members manage conflict effectively instead of avoiding it.	5	4	3	2	1	U/A
Learners are integrated into the team.	5	4	3	2	1	U/A
The patient is integrated into the team.	5	4	3	2	1	U/A
Team members take time to reflect on how to improve patient care.	5	4	3	2	1	U/A

Source: Wendy S. Madigosky, M.D., M.S.P.H., University of Colorado School of Medicine, 2006.

TABLE 3-3.

Roles and Relative Involvement in Care by Each Health Care Professional for Specific Cases*

Health Care Professional	Patient Case Example			
	18-Year-Old Female with a Fractured Femur from a Motor Vehicle Accident	77-Year-Old Male with Metastatic Lung Cancer Receiving Hospice Care at Home	65-Year-Old Female with Stable Atrial Fibrillation Taking Warfarin Daily	42-Year-Old Male Without Health Insurance Who Requires a Kidney Transplant
Physician	XXX	X	X	XX
Nurse	XX	XXX	X	XX
Pharmacist	XX	XX	XXX	XX
Health care administrator	X	XX	X	XXX

* X = minimal involvement, XX = moderate involvement, XXX = substantial involvement. This table shows relative estimates based on knowledge of the focus of care for each individual patient. Understanding the relative role in each setting is important in identifying members of an improvement team and understanding the insight from each health care professional.

Summary

Working in teams is necessary for efficient and effective improvement work. As a health professional, your clinical and technical expertise will be invaluable for improvement work. Improvement work also requires leadership from and the participation of other health care professionals. Having a basic understanding of their background and training is important. To lead improvement efforts, you must know how to organize an interprofessional team and assess its effectiveness. And to be an excellent team member, you must know when to defer to the expertise of other health care professionals. With the goal of improved patient care—and a reliable system to deliver that care—patients and their families deserve no less than our full attention to effective teamwork across all professions.

Study Questions

1. Consider a time when you were part of a health care team—a time, perhaps, when you shadowed a physician during a clinical rotation. Now think of patients you saw during that experience who were particularly complex, such as ambulatory patients with difficult-to-control diabetes, colon surgery patients with several comorbidities, or children with chronic diseases such as cystic fibrosis.
   a. Write a description of the setting and population.
   b. Complete a row in the following table for each team member who contributed to the care of these patients. The first row is completed as an example to help you get started. Be sure to consider team members who may not have directly interacted with the patients but did influence their care.

Team Member	Professional Role	Work Duties on the Team
Kim Yoon	*Physician*	*Diagnosing and recommending treatment for patient*
		Offering emotional support to patient and family

2. Review the team list you created. Was this the right mix of professionals to care for this group of patients? Why or why not? What would have made the team stronger?

3. Did you include patients and families as part of the care team? Discuss whether patients and families should routinely be included as part of the care team.

References

1. Katzenbach J.R., Smith D.K.: The discipline of teams. *Harvard Business Review*, The Best of HBR 1993, Jul.–Aug. 2005, 1–9.

2. Scholtes P.R., Joiner B.L., Streibel B.J.: *The Team Handbook*, 3rd ed. Madison, WI: Oriel Inc., 2003.

3. Headrick L.A., et al.: *Module 2: Build a Team.* Healthcare Improvement Skills Center. http://www.improvementskills.com (accessed Jan. 24, 2008).

4. Batalden P.B., et al.: Microsystems in health care: Part 9. Developing small clinical units to attain peak performance. *Jt Comm J Qual Patient Saf* 29:575–585, Nov. 2003.

5. Weinstein J.N., et al.: Designing an ambulatory clinical practice for outcomes improvement: From vision to reality—The Spine Center at Dartmouth-Hitchcock, year one. *Qual Manag Health Care* 8:1–20, Winter 2000.

6. Oandasan I., Reeves S.C.: Key elements for interprofessional education. Part 1: The learner, the educator and the learning context. *J Interprof Care*, 19(suppl.1):2, 21–38, May 1, 2005 (accessed Aug. 11, 2009).

7. Health Professions Networks, Nursing & Midwifery, Human Resources for Health: *Framework for Action on Interprofessional Education & Collaborative Practice.* Geneva: World Health Organization, 2010. http://whqlibdoc.who.int/hq/2010/WHO_HRH_HPN_10.3_eng.pdf (accessed May 19, 2011).

8. Interprofessional Education Collaborative Expert Panel: *Core Competencies for Interprofessional Collaborative Practice: Report of an Expert Panel.* Washington, DC: Interprofessional Education Collaborative, 2011.

9. Greiner A.C., Knebel E. (eds.), Institute of Medicine: *Health Professions Education: A Bridge to Quality.* Washington, DC: National Academies Press, 2003.

10. Cronenwett L., et al.: Quality and safety education for nurses. *Nurs Outlook* 55:122–131, May–Jun., 2007.

11. Beckett C.D., Kipnis G.: Collaborative communication: Integrating SBAR to improve quality/patient safety outcomes. *J Healthc Qual* 31:19–28, Sep.–Oct. 2009.

12. Haig K.M., Sutton S., Whittington J.: SBAR: A shared mental model for improving communication between clinicians. *Jt Comm J Qual Patient Saf* 32:167–175, Mar. 2006.

13. McCarthy D., Chase D.: Advancing patient safety in the U.S. Department of Veterans Affairs. *The Commonwealth Fund* 9, Mar. 15, 2011. http://www.commonwealthfund.org/Content/Publications/Case-Studies/2011/Mar/Advancing-Patient-Safety.aspx (accessed May 19, 2011).

14. Agency for Healthcare Research and Quality: *About TeamSTEPPS.* http://teamstepps.ahrq.gov/about-2cl_3.htm (accessed May 19, 2011).

15. Sexton J.B., Thomas E.J., Helmreich R.L.: Error, stress, and teamwork in medicine and aviation: Cross sectional surveys. *BMJ* 320:745–749, Mar. 18, 2000.

CHAPTER 4

Targeting an Improvement Effort

OBJECTIVES

After reading this chapter, you will be able to do the following:

1. Identify areas of a system that need to be improved, informed by knowledge of the needs of the people to be served.
2. State ways to narrow the focus of improvement work.
3. Write an aim statement for improvement that is specific, measurable, attainable, and reasonable and has a time frame (S.M.A.R.T.).

Maria Martinez, a first-year medical resident, looks puzzled. She is sitting at a conference room table with the attending physician, the nurse practitioner, and a few members of the clinic's quality improvement team. They are discussing possibilities for improving the continuity of care at the free clinic where they all work. Maria is puzzled because she has spent considerable time thinking about something to improve for her residency requirements, but when she discusses the possibilities with the team and her attending physician, Phil Morrison, she is overwhelmed. Maria looks at the attending and then at the whiteboard that lists possible improvement projects. Finally, she asks, "How can we decide? There are too many things that need to be improved, and I just don't know where to start."

Phil turns to the board, reviews the list aloud, and says, "Which of these is most important to the patient population we serve: patient waiting time, evidence-based treatment of urinary tract infections, diabetes care, preventive services, or the reporting of x-ray findings to patients? We have a long list, but we need to start somewhere. Let's look at our data to determine the greatest patient needs and then ask ourselves, 'What bothers us the most?'"

Maria obtains some of the quality data from the clinic and realizes that there are big gaps in providing primary prevention. She knows that this is an important aspect to the population she serves, as these interventions prevent disease from ever starting. In the first six months of her residency training, she tried to use a template for preventive care, but her template left her frustrated. She realizes that the lack of preventive care delivered is an area that bothers her the most. Dave Thomas, an advanced practice nurse practitioner, has cautioned Maria about the lack of time available to address preventive care problems during a scheduled visit. Dave suggests that a team approach consistent with a patient medical home model may be the answer. Maria turns to the attending and says, "I'd really like to improve disease prevention for patients in our clinic." "Great! Identifying something in our system that needs to be improved is the first step," he replies. "The next steps are to focus that idea and then to create an aim statement. We will discuss ways to focus your idea when we meet again later this week."

An integral component of improving health care is to target the improvement efforts. The Model for Improvement (*see* Figure 4-1 below) is a useful guide to ensure success of these efforts. This chapter addresses the first question in the Model for Improvement: "What are we trying to accomplish?" To answer this question, it is helpful to go through a three-step process:

1. Identify a general area to improve.
2. Narrow the focus.
3. Create an aim statement to guide the project.

FIGURE 4-1. *The Model for Improvement*

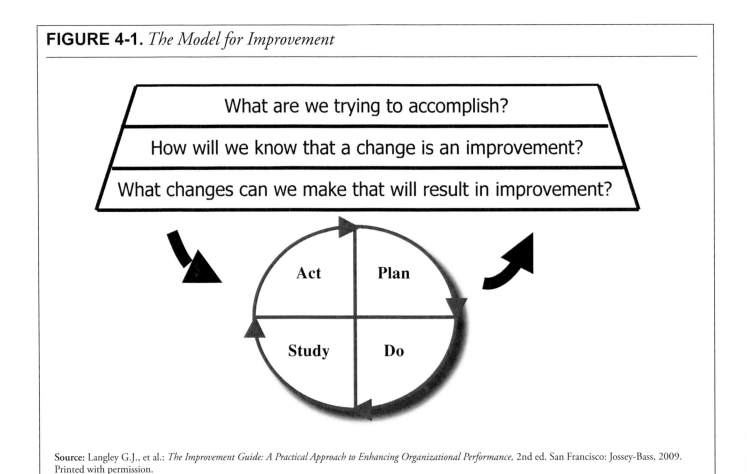

Source: Langley G.J., et al.: *The Improvement Guide: A Practical Approach to Enhancing Organizational Performance,* 2nd ed. San Francisco: Jossey-Bass, 2009. Printed with permission.

Sidebar 4-1. *Pushing System Performance to the Theoretical Limit*

Setting the goal in an aim statement almost always involves a numeric goal, such as "25% increase in *X*," "decrease *Y* by 50%," or "improve the rate of *Z* from 62% to 85%." Targets such as these are very helpful. These types of targets provide clear goals for a team; however, why aim for only a 25% change or to reach 85%? In order to provide the right care to the right patient at the right time, shouldn't the target be 100%? When a goal is set at the absolute best, it is referred to as the *theoretical limit* of performance.

The *theoretical limit* is defined as the performance of a system that is *possible*. "Possible" is the key consideration and is differentiated from "probable." The "probable" performance is the likely level of performance that has been reported by others, perhaps in a journal article, as a best practice at a conference, or through benchmarking. The theoretical limit is reached by asking, "What if we were able to achieve 100% performance?" or "How could we achieve a 0% error rate?" This can be a powerful frame of mind to push system performance to higher levels. Sometimes, the incremental goal is the appropriate one; sometimes, the theoretical limit is the appropriate goal.

In 2004 the Institute for Healthcare Improvement (IHI) started a campaign in the United States to save 100,000 lives through the widespread implementation of five evidence-based interventions for hospitalized patients: deploy rapid response teams for patients with declining clinical conditions, provide reliable care for patients with acute myocardial infarctions, provide medication reconciliation to prevent medication errors, decrease ventilator-associated pneumonia (VAP), and decrease central venous catheter infections.[1] At the start of the 100,000 Lives Campaign, some in health care assumed that some of these conditions were inevitable for a certain percentage of hospitalized patients. It was not uncommon for an intubated patient on mechanical ventilation to develop pneumonia. Also, because central venous catheter use is common in critically ill patients in intensive care units, many assumed that a certain percentage of these patients would develop these infections. More than 2,500 hospitals in the United States joined the 100,000 Lives Campaign, and most set goals for incremental decreases in their rates of VAP and central venous catheter infections.

Over time, many hospitals involved in the 100,000 Lives Campaign decreased their rates of both VAP and central line infections by using standard, bundled, evidence-based interventions. In 2007 the IHI followed up with the participating hospitals. It found nearly 50 hospitals that had gone more than two years without a single case of VAP and about 40 hospitals that had gone more than two years without a single central line infection. These sites had set the theoretical limit as their goal. They were not satisfied with incremental improvement (although perhaps they started with incremental goals), and they pushed the systems to higher performance, with these infections driven to zero—the absolute best. They entered a new state of balance, where patients are not expected to get these infections at all, for at these hospitals an infection is an unusual occurrence.

It is important to consider the theoretical limit when setting goals. Is a 90% outcome really good enough? Should a site be satisfied with a 50% or 60% decrease in bloodstream infections? Using the theoretical limit can push a team to consider the best possible performance—the level of commitment that patients and their families deserve.

Step 1: Identifying an Improvement Area

So how do you find potential areas to improve? One way is to start by looking at the systems you are a part of. As you will learn in Chapter 5, a *system* is a set of interdependent elements working together to achieve a common aim. These elements may be both human and nonhuman (for example, technology, equipment, information). Even as a student, you are a part of many systems: a personal system with a pattern of eating, sleeping, exercising, and studying; an educational system of clinical groups, lab groups, and study groups; and clinical care systems, such as those in a nursing clinical rotation or a medical clerkship. In each of these systems, you interact with various people, processes, and structures. While the focus of this book is on creating improvement in clinical systems, identifying opportunities and practicing improvement skills in personal and educational systems can be a practical way to gain experience with improvement skills.

As a student, you likely see processes within the system that could be improved. For example, within your school, such processes might include student career counseling or the way clinical rotations are assigned. In addition, students may see opportunities for improving processes in the clinical system. One first-year medical student stated, "When I started at my preceptor's office back in August, I said, 'Wow, this is spectacular.' After working there for eight months, I recognized how many processes in the clinical system could be improved. The patients had long wait times and often had to call back for clarification of medications." A fourth-year nursing student, in his clinical rotation on an orthopedic floor, found that care was not always consistent with the evidence-based practice of turning patients every two hours to prevent pressure ulcers. The nursing student knew this was important both clinically and financially, as hospitals would no longer be reimbursed for any hospital-acquired pressure ulcers. Anywhere systems and processes exist, they can be improved, and identifying opportunities to improve is an important first step.

Identifying improvement areas in clinical care requires that you reflect on the care delivered, viewing it through an "improvement lens" of mindfulness (being aware of how your practice is impacting the patient) and system thinking (looking beyond what you do and considering all the factors that impact the quality of your patient care). Improvement areas can be identified in your personal performance within the clinical care system as well as at the micro- and macrosystem levels of practice. While it is easy to think about personal performance areas for improvement, identifying improvement areas at the clinical system level is more difficult.

Approaches to Identifying Improvement Areas

The following approaches will help you identify an improvement area at the system level:

- **Examine point-of-care issues.** At the system level, think about what you see in practice. Are there any procedures being carried out that do not follow policy? Are there gaps between evidence-based practice and what you see happening every day?

- **Review data.** Opportunities for improvement must be informed by knowledge of the needs of the people served. The best way to examine these needs is to use data that are often collected for regulatory requirements. In the acute care setting, for example, each unit has data that indicate the quality of care delivered; unit- and hospital-level data are available for many issues, such as pressure ulcers, falls, infections, and incident reports. Satisfaction scores and feedback summaries are also available and may help point you toward improvement opportunities.
- **Discuss and reflect on frustrations.** Still another way ideas may arise is from discussions with colleagues about their frustrations with the system. To identify an improvement area, frequently all you need to do is ask yourself, "What is the one process that frustrates me the most?" Often your frustrations reflect the needs of the patients you serve.

These approaches likely will produce many potential improvement ideas. It is important to prioritize the list you generate by considering the population served, best practices, and the greatest patient needs.

After you have identified the general area in which you would like to make improvements (for example, ensuring evidence-based treatment of urinary tract infection), the second step is to narrow the focus.

Step 2: Narrowing the Focus of the Improvement Work

Maria, the first-year medical resident, mulls over this question: "Given what I've learned about how our clinic is doing, what is most frustrating to me about preventive care in the free clinic?" She is aware that the care in the free clinic is a team effort that includes the patient and many professionals: administrative assistants, medical assistants, nurses, and clinical provider colleagues (that is, other resident physicians, nurse practitioners, and attending physicians). She has a conversation in the hallway with Dave Thomas, the nurse practitioner, and Nick Borysenko, a medical assistant. The three of them briefly review the work of all the team members. As the medical assistant, Nick obtains the chief complaint, triages the urgency of the visit, and takes the vital signs. The nurse practitioner is an independent clinician who has a primary care panel in the same clinic as the intern. They are all frustrated about the difficulty in providing healthy living guidance to patients. In the limited time allotted for appointments, there are important prevention topics—such as diet modification, exercise counseling, and tobacco avoidance—that they often are not able to cover in any great depth.

Dave and Nick share Maria's passion to provide counseling on healthy living for all the patients in the clinic. The team members agree that this is an important goal for an improvement project; diet and exercise counseling do not get enough emphasis in care providers' time with patients. Phil, who works as an attending physician in other clinics, says to the group, "Hmm. That's helpful to hear that you all find this to be an issue. Tell me about the template for healthy living that you currently use. How much information is on it?"

Maria tells the group about the three main parts of her preventive medicine template: (1) guidelines for preventive treatments such as vaccinations, (2) screening information for services such as mammograms and colonoscopies, and (3) healthy living counseling, including diet and exercise guidance. Nick points out that healthy living counseling is the responsibility of the clinic's providers and that the preventive guidelines and screening are standardized for the whole clinic. Dave has his own healthy living counseling approach, which he has developed over his 12 years as a nurse practitioner. Nick states, "Almost all the providers have a healthy living counseling approach . . . and they're all different."

Maria sums it up: "All right, so this is simple. Our focus will be to 'improve the healthy living counseling for the patients at the medical center clinic.'" Phil, looking thoughtful, says, "Well . . . we're getting closer. You've done a great job of narrowing the focus. When we meet next, we will address the third step—that is, to craft a clear aim that will guide the entire project."

As we saw in the opening vignette, Maria Martinez is frustrated with the range and number of opportunities that she sees need improvement in the clinic. Like many other professionals, she's finding it difficult to narrow what she wants to improve and feels overwhelmed by wanting to improve everything. It's important to narrow the focus. For example, an improvement team might begin with the goal of improving care for patients with diabetes in a primary care practice, including glycemic control, hypertension, and lifestyle changes. While each of these is worthy of the team's attention, creating an improvement project that is too broad is a common pitfall. A team that doesn't appropriately narrow the focus of its goals may endure many iterations and travel several paths without ever achieving real improvement in any area. This leads to wandering work, unclear priorities, and frustration.

A team that doesn't appropriately narrow the focus of its goals may endure many iterations and travel several paths without ever achieving real improvement in any area.

Criteria to Focus Improvement Goals

If you've done research, you've learned how important it is to narrow the focus of a research question. Hulley and colleagues describe a strong research question as having five characteristics: *feasible, interesting, novel, ethical,* and *relevant (FINER).*[2] We can use these criteria to focus improvement goals. Although research and quality improvement are different in implementation and execution, they both share the common goal of generating new information, and both are potential opportunities for students to publish with their mentors. The FINER characteristics will be addressed shortly, in the context of quality improvement work, in order to narrow the focus.

Feasible. Your improvement project should be *feasible* within the practical limits of your position. A project that you choose to do as a student might be very different from a project you would lead as an attending physician or a registered nurse. As you study this book, the improvement methodology you learn will form a foundation for years to come. The results of your work can be equally satisfying, but the feasibility of the project must match with your current position and authority to act within your professional discipline.

Interesting. The topic for an improvement project should be *interesting* to you and to your organization. If you are working on a personal improvement project, you should be passionate about the topic. For example, it may be important for you to work on something you have experienced as problematic, such as on-time starts for patient appointments or remembering to wash hands. If a group of students are working to improve an educational topic, they should check with the school administration to see what's on the radar. For example, a team of students at Dartmouth Medical School was interested in increasing the availability of career counseling for first- and second-year students. By coincidence, the medical school was preparing for a site visit by the Liaison Committee on Medical Education (LCME) from the Association of American Medical Colleges (AAMC) in the coming months. The medical students' interest in this project was of vital importance to them as students. The analysis that they performed was important for them, for their classmates, and also for the school because it helped with the LCME report and site visit. This was a win–win situation for the students (analyzing and improving the system of career counseling for first- and second-year medical students) and for the medical school (demonstrating evidence of student involvement in improving the student experience for the LCME site visitors).

Novel. An improvement project should be *novel.* In Chapter 1, we discussed the fact that improvement work is the act of implementing the best practice in a local setting. Improvement work generally does not generate new, generalizable knowledge in the same way that research does, but it provides an opportunity to learn about local systems and make changes that are important to the people served by those systems. Improvement work will generate new local knowledge about a system, and it allows you to optimize the performance and outcomes of local processes, whether the project involves improving preceptorships for fourth-year nursing students or increasing the use of appropriate antibiotics for patients with pneumonia.

Ethical. Your improvement project should be *ethical.* This is an essential up-front consideration when choosing a project. There should be assurances that the project poses no threat of physical or psychological harm to individuals and that there will be no invasion of privacy. It is important to have early consultation with local improvement project sponsors to determine whether Institutional Review Board (IRB) review is required. An IRB is a committee designated to approve, monitor, and review research to protect the rights and welfare of research subjects, and this committee has the authority to determine whether quality improvement work should be considered research. IRB practices may differ somewhat from institution to institution, and a thorough review by the Hastings Center in 2006 showed that most current institutional IRBs are ill prepared to evaluate improvement projects.[3] Since that report was published, IRBs have instituted policies to examine the ethical issues surrounding quality improvement projects. Although improvement work and research share many characteristics, improvement of care is integral to the delivery of care; therefore, the protection of patients during improvement activities should be part of a transformed system of accountability in clinical care. Remember to consult with professionals who

DEFINED: IRB
An IRB is a committee designated to approve, monitor, and review research to protect the rights and welfare of research subjects, and this committee has the authority to determine whether quality improvement work should be considered research.

IRB practices may differ somewhat from institution to institution, and a thorough review by the Hastings Center in 2006 showed that most current institutional IRBs are ill prepared to evaluate improvement projects.

have improvement experience to help guide the team through the local improvement process, including when to involve the local IRB.

Relevant. An improvement project needs to be *relevant*. For clinical improvement projects, it is important that the topic be relevant to patients, staff, and administration. For example, the U.S. Veterans Health Administration (VHA), a component of the U.S. Department of Veterans Affairs (VA), commenced a large improvement effort across 40 institutions to reduce falls and injuries due to falls in hospitalized patients.[4] The VHA—both nationally and also from local VA hospitals—committed funding, personnel, and support for the improvement work. Patient falls are high-profile events for patients and families, and injuries from falls (such as hip fractures or head injuries) can add increased length of stay and costs to a patient's hospitalization.[5] This issue was of high importance to the patients, to the individual VA hospitals, and to the national VA. Each facility identified a passionate, interprofessional work group that consisted of physicians, nurses, physical therapists, and occupational therapists. This example demonstrates how a focus of improvement (reducing falls and injury due to falls) is relevant for all stakeholders in the organization—patients, families, clinicians, administrators—at both local and national levels. Tight alignment of priorities—those of patients, providers, hospitals, and the national VA—was an important element for keeping this project relevant and reducing falls.

Step 3: Creating an Aim Statement

After narrowing the focus of the improvement work, your third step is to create an aim statement. Starting improvement work without a clear aim statement is akin to conducting research without a clear hypothesis. Absence of clear direction often leads to wasted time and effort. A clear aim will keep a project on track, help identify the process, and aid in identifying proper measures. Now that we have discussed some of the characteristics of finding a project and narrowing the focus, we'll try to put it all together by developing an aim statement. Let us return to our scenario to discover what a clear aim for a project looks like.

The improvement team reflects on its progress. Nick Borysenko and Maria Martinez agree that this project is doable and would be of interest to many in primary care. Although this project would not be particularly novel for the clinic, it would serve an important need for the patients, and, if successful, it would be very useful for other clinics, too. No one can identify any ethical concerns with this project.

Maria leads the team to focus the thinking: "So we started with this goal: 'Improve the healthy living counseling for the patients at the medical center clinic.' This is a reasonable start, but because the aim statement is going to be a guiding statement for the project, the content of the aim should completely represent the project. Will we improve healthy living counseling for all patients in the clinic?" Nick replies, "It would be quite a feat to work with all the patients! We have at least a dozen providers, nurses, and administrative assistants. Perhaps our first efforts should involve only a few practitioners."

Dave Thomas agrees and says, "Because we all have such a strong interest in this, perhaps we could start with something like this: 'Over the next six months, we will improve the delivery of information regarding the benefits of diet and exercise for primary prevention for our patients.'" Refining the aim has helped the group feel like it has a clear direction. The team members realize that much work needs to be done, but this step was necessary to get started.

As our scenario continues to unfold, we see how Phil Morrison, the attending, is able to coach the team to develop a specific aim from an initial general interest in preventive care, dig deeper into the issues surrounding the delivery of preventive medicine, test the feasibility and relevance of the project, and create a clear and concise aim statement. The team is now positioned to use its aim statement as a clear guide for developing measures (described in Chapter 6) and identifying interventions to test change (discussed in Chapter 8) in the clinic system.

Using S.M.A.R.T. Criteria to Define a Clear Aim Statement

In many ways, the aim statement for an improvement project reads like the first sentence of a newspaper article. In one sentence of a newspaper article, you know *what* happened *where*, *who* was involved, *when* it occurred, and perhaps even *how* it transpired. The aim for improvement work should be equally descriptive.

Components of an effective aim statement can be described with the S.M.A.R.T. criteria.[6] The first criterion is that an aim needs to be *specific* (S) and can be sharpened by including the who, what, where, when, and why components. Next, an aim needs to be *measurable* (M) and include concrete criteria for assessing progress toward attainment of the goal. The aim should also be *attainable* (A) and *reasonable* (R), and it must represent an objective that is achievable and that you are willing and able to work toward. Finally, an aim needs to be grounded within a *time frame* (T).

Here is an example to illustrate the components of a S.M.A.R.T. aim. A group of nursing students on a clinical rotation observed that the date of intravenous (IV) tubing initiation was not being marked. They knew that tubing needed to be changed every three days, per hospital protocol. Because the tubing was not marked with a date of initiation, the students were unsure when to change the tubing. They formed a quality improvement team with the staff on the unit and proposed this aim statement: "By the end of our clinical rotation, 100% of the IV tubing will be marked with the date that the tubing was initiated and changed." This aim statement follows the S.M.A.R.T. criteria: specific (IV tubing will be marked with start and changed dates), measureable (100% marked tubing), attainable, reasonable, and timely (by the end of the clinical rotation).

To differentiate what is a clear aim, we provide examples of aims developed by teams working to decrease falls and injuries due to falls (*see* Table 4-1 on page 52). The first example is not a strong aim. The team certainly gets credit for being honest, but the locus of control is outside the team ("clinical manager"), and the goal is not very clear.

S.M.A.R.T.

S = *Specific*
M = *Measurable*
A = *Attainable*
R = *Reasonable*
T = *Time frame*

TABLE 4-1.

Examples of Aim Statements for Reducing Falls in Hospitalized Patients

Sample Aim	Characteristics
Unclear Aim: Our clinical manager directed us to reduce falls in patients.	• Identifies main purpose • Has a locus of incentive that is external to the team • Does not include a time frame or a measurable goal
Unclear Aim: On ward 2-South, reduce patient falls over the next week.	• Contains clear description of the location of the improvement work • Has a time frame that is not reasonable or attainable • Does not include a measurable goal or a description of the team
Clear Aim: Working with the falls reduction team on ward 2-South, we will reduce the rate of patient falls by 25% over the next six months.	• Is a very clear aim that meets S.M.A.R.T. criteria (specific, measurable, attainable, and reasonable and has a time frame)

The second example is slightly better because it contains a defined location ("2-South") as well as a time frame ("one week"); however, the goal is not clearly defined, and the time frame is not reasonable.

The third example is an aim that is specific and concise and meets the S.M.A.R.T. criteria. It tells the specifics of the project (exactly who will be working on this project and where they will focus), the desired measurable outcome ("reduce by 25%"), and a time frame to guide the project ("in the next six months"). The aim also is attainable and reasonable as stated. A stated time frame is an important element when chartering a quality improvement project. Stating a time frame gives a clear message to all involved that this is not a team that will stagnate but one that will reevaluate its goals at reasonable intervals. This final example will serve the team well as it starts making changes on 2-South. It will help to refocus the team as data roll in and the team evaluates whether any of the changes have led to improvements in care. Clear aim statements are vital for the success of any improvement project, whether it is a personal project, an educational project, or a clinical project.

Summary

Determining an area for improvement work is not always simple. While there are many opportunities in health care to do improvement work, we must always be mindful of the needs of the people we serve. The three steps discussed in this chapter—identifying an improvement opportunity, narrowing the focus, and creating a S.M.A.R.T. aim—provide a framework to help us answer the first question in the Model for Improvement: "What are we trying to accomplish?"[7] Creating a clear and focused aim statement during the planning of an improvement project will save time and energy downstream and also will keep the project focused as it moves forward. The aim statement serves as a summary of and a compass for the project.

Study Questions
Identifying Opportunities for Improvement

Each of the following scenarios describes either an educational or a clinical situation that is in need of improvement. There may be several aspects of the situation that need to be improved. After you read each scenario, determine where you might focus your improvement efforts and describe your reasoning.

Scenario 1

As you complete your first six months as a medical student at your preceptor's office, you reflect on what a wonderful experience it has been. You get plenty of time to see patients on your own, and your preceptor even observes some part of your interview and/or examination at every session. You have been fully integrated into the practice, and sometimes you even arrive early on your preceptor day to attend the lunchtime practice meeting. It seems like a good way to grab a bite to eat and learn about how this small, rural practice operates.

At this month's practice meeting, the office secretary is concerned about a recent decrease in the availability of urgent care appointments. The nurse states that it seems that several appointments per week are used for women who complain of pain and burning with urination. Your preceptor explains that these visits are necessary to evaluate the possibility of a kidney infection and to determine the proper antibiotic regimen for the suspected urinary tract infection. You recall reading an article about using a nurse triage protocol on the phone to treat simple urinary tract infections. Your preceptor would like your input on how to address this problem.

- What can you suggest to get this started? Why would you suggest this plan? What would be your aim?

Scenario 2

You are a nursing student doing a clinical rotation on a general medical floor. Your patient is a 60-year-old male with type 2 diabetes admitted for the third time this year with hyperglycemia. The physician is frustrated because he has been working very hard to improve this patient's glycemic control. The patient continues to be in poor control;

his most recent hemoglobin A1C was 9.3% (normal is less than 6%). You talk with the patient, and you find that he is overwhelmed by having to make so many lifestyle changes. You decide to use your improvement skills and develop with the patient an aim statement using the S.M.A.R.T. criteria. The patient shares that he mostly struggles with doing finger sticks at home.

- What would the aim statement be in this scenario?

Identifying and Evaluating the Components of an Aim Statement

For each of the following clinical improvement scenarios, indicate whether the aim statement is consistent with the S.M.A.R.T. criteria (specific, measurable, attainable, realistic, timely). If it does not meet one or more of these, then state how the aim could be improved to include more or all of the criteria.

Scenario 1

Gosia Nichols is a third-year medical resident in obstetrics and gynecology. Many patients who are only a few weeks pregnant will present to the clinic with vaginal bleeding. This is commonly termed a miscarriage, or an incomplete spontaneous abortion. Although this is a relatively common presenting condition, Gosia has been frustrated. She has recognized that the treatment that is recommended for this condition depends on who is the attending in the clinic that day. Some attending physicians prefer medical management, some prefer surgical management, and some prefer watchful waiting. Gosia uses her practice-based learning and improvement four-week rotation to develop a plan to address this issue. After reviewing the literature and identifying the evidence-based guidelines for treatment of incomplete spontaneous abortions, she prepares an aim for her work.

Aim: Over the next 24 months, we will increase the use of evidence-based treatment by 25% for first-trimester incomplete spontaneous abortions at the residents' clinic.

- Write an improved aim statement for this scenario.

Scenario 2

Throughout his first year in nursing school, Fadi Mathias has been frustrated by the students' use of information technology. He worked for an Internet company before coming to nursing school and knows that wikis, listservs, and blogs could help the students communicate more effectively. Currently, most of the students (as well as faculty and administration) use only e-mail to communicate. Fadi would like to develop a free online community for his classmates, but he is not sure which online tools would be used the most. He teams up with several other students and a faculty leader, and they chart a course to address this issue.

Aim: Through the use of focus groups and a survey, identify and implement online community tools for first-year students.

- Write an improved aim statement for this scenario.

Scenario 3

Since John Fariq began medical school, he has wanted to complete a residency in orthopedic surgery. Now that he has the opportunity to do a sub-internship, John is very excited to make a good impression. Although he enjoys the excitement of the operating room, he finds evaluating patients in the orthopedic clinic less interesting. Through the first 10 days of this rotation, he is particularly bothered by how often the x-rays are not available for the team in the clinic. This creates delays and frustrations for the patients and the staff as the right information (x-ray) is not available to make decisions for patients. Sometimes when an x-ray cannot be retrieved, the patient is sent for a repeat x-ray film. This is wasteful to all. John decides to help solve this problem and presents an aim statement to his faculty preceptor.

Aim: Working with the orthopedic clinic staff, we will decrease the rate of missing x-rays by 50% over the next three weeks.

- Write an improved aim statement for this scenario.

Analyzing Ethical Considerations of Improvement Work

For each of the following scenarios, describe the ethical challenge that should be addressed.

Scenario 1

Ed Stepstein was excited to be working on a project to improve the safety of unfractionated heparin use in the intensive care unit (ICU). As a fourth-year nursing student, he had some experience with the considerable variability in the partial thromboplastin times (PTTs) of patients treated with unfractionated heparin. His quality improvement (QI) elective was an opportunity to work with a team in the ICU to show how few patients had therapeutic PTTs. Ed spent several hours at one of the computer work stations at the hospital, reviewing charts and lab results. He created a comprehensive database that listed the patients, the dates of admission, and the PTT lab values for all patients treated with unfractionated heparin in the past 12 months. He was anxious to begin the analysis, so he copied the file to his thumb drive and headed home to continue his work after dinner on his home computer.

- What cause for concern does this scenario illustrate?
  (Answer: Patients' personal health information must be kept private. Data collected for QI must be held to the same standards of privacy as any other personal health information. Transferring data to a thumb drive and to a personal computer puts these data at risk. The data should either be stored on a secure server at the hospital or should be de-identified.)

Scenario 2

Ana Zamar is excited about being a first-year internal medicine resident and developing her own patient panel. She enjoys the relationship building and physician–

patient interactions that occur over time. She feels fortunate to have attended a medical school that emphasizes practice-based learning and improvement and systems-based practice, and she believes she is ready to build and improve care for her patients. Having just heard about a new diabetes medication that was recently released, Ana writes a clear aim (with the S.M.A.R.T. criteria to guide her work). She sets up a small electronic database of her patients who have diabetes and sends out a letter to every other patient on the list, informing them that they will be starting on this new medication. She is excited to track the results and see if the new medication improves diabetes outcomes for her patients.

- What cause for concern does this scenario illustrate?

(Answer: This is closer to a research project than a QI project. Assigning a new drug to half the patients without tailoring the treatment is not applying best evidence to patients. There are many choices for diabetes medications, and those treatment options need to be chosen for each individual patient. Also, Ana is testing a new medication in a group of patients without first obtaining their consent to do so.)

References

1. Berwick D.M., et al.: The 100,000 Lives Campaign: Setting a goal and a deadline for improving health care quality. *JAMA* 295:324–327, Jan. 18, 2006.
2. Hulley S.B., et al.: *Designing Clinical Research*, 2nd ed. Philadelphia: Lippincott, Williams & Wilkins, 2001.
3. Baily M.A., et al.: The ethics of using QI methods to improve health care quality and safety. *Hastings Cent Rep* 36:S1–S40, Jul.–Aug. 2006.
4. Mills P.D., et al.: Reducing falls and fall-related injuries in the VA system. *Journal of Health Care Safety Quarterly* 1:25–33, Winter 2003.
5. Oliver D., et al.: Risk factors and risk assessment tools for falls in hospital in-patients: A systematic review. *Age Ageing* 33:122–130, Mar. 2004.
6. Doran, G.T.: There's a S.M.A.R.T. way to write management's goals and objectives. *Manage Rev* 70:35–36, 1981.
7. Langley G.J., et al.: *The Improvement Guide: A Practical Approach to Enhancing Organizational Performance*, 2nd ed. San Francisco: Jossey-Bass, 2009.

CHAPTER 5

Process Literacy

OBJECTIVES

After reading this chapter, you will be able to do the following:

1. Recognize the importance of describing the process of care that is being studied.
2. Identify how the process of care is related to the context of care.
3. Select from a variety of process modeling methods to describe patient care scenarios, including brainstorming and using cause-and-effect diagrams, flow diagrams, deployment flowcharts, and workflow diagrams.

"Big changes are planned." That's the buzz in the clinic as nurse practitioner Selena Delacruz and physician James Simon arrive to cover their shifts in the drop-in clinic. The drop-in clinic is the place for acute medical needs at the medical center—a step below the emergency department in patient acuity. No appointments are necessary; the clinic gives a patient the opportunity to show up and be evaluated for any general medical concern. Selena and James discover that the drop-in clinic is going to switch from being a "no appointment necessary" clinic to being an "appointments only" clinic. "This should be interesting," they both muse.

James settles in for what's sure to be a long afternoon. He looks at the cart piled high with patient charts. As each patient arrives at the clinic, he or she is checked in and triaged by a nurse before his or her chart is placed at the bottom of the stack. Clinicians then pull charts from the top of the stack to see patients in the order in which they arrived. James has been working at the clinic for six months and has never thought this system worked well, but the process was already in place when he started there. He needs to be at the clinic only a half day per week, and he finds it easiest to go with the current flow. Selena, however, was one of the developers of the current process (which was thought to be highly innovative at the time). She is skeptical about the proposed change and thinks it may not have been properly planned.

Changes will be coming, however. The department formed a committee that recommended that all patients have appointments in order to be seen in this clinic. No one is quite sure how the new process will operate. James is not even sure how the current process is operating;

he wonders whether the new process will replace the current one or serve as an alternative to it. Selena is really comfortable with the current system, although she acknowledges that it has drawbacks at times. As James and Selena grab their first charts for the afternoon, each notices the huge crowd of patients in the waiting room. They see that the front-desk workers are scrambling to get patients checked in. And in the triage room, the nurses are busy assessing the severity of each patient's chief complaint. As they take all this in, James and Selena wonder just how well the patients' acute care needs are being met here at the medical center.

Process Analysis

Many processes are embedded in health care. Processes in health care are not inherently good or bad, but each has developed for a reason. Sometimes a process develops because it is the most efficient way to provide care to patients; sometimes processes develop because of patient or family feedback; some processes exist because they are convenient for billing purposes; and some processes help an organization comply with rules and regulations.

DEFINED:
Process Illiteracy
and Process Arrogance

Process illiteracy is a lack of familiarity with what actually happens, day-to-day, from the patient's point of view. Process arrogance is an exaggerated sense of knowing how things work.

Although all providers are part of these systems and processes, they are often process illiterate. *Process illiteracy* is a lack of familiarity with what actually happens, day-to-day, from the patient's point of view. Perhaps even more concerning is *process arrogance*—an exaggerated sense of knowing how things work. Many feel that they know processes because they work in the environment. But systems are complex. Process arrogance is usually not a deliberate decision, but rather it is a sense that develops over time due to exposure to routines. Because health care processes tend to be complex interactions among clinicians, administrators, patients, families, information, and technology, no one person can fully experience health care processes from all vantage points. Knowledge of the structures, patterns, and people within a system begins to demonstrate process literacy and is a vital step in the improvement of systems.

The Importance of Process Analysis

Why is knowing a process and how it operates important for the improvement of care? Process analysis—including the measurement of key steps of the process—is crucial to improvement for three reasons.

Process analysis provides a common picture—a shared model—for an improvement team. Each member of the team experiences processes differently. The administrative staff, the front-desk staff, nurses, physicians, medical assistants, and the pharmacist all have information about what actually occurs. Describing the process of care from the patient and family's point of view with input from all the stakeholders—including patients and families—creates a shared model, one that can be used and understood by everyone. This model is an important tool for keeping the patient experience at the center of the conversation about improvement.

Process analysis helps identify which parts of the system are important to measure in order to understand and improve the care system. When a process is depicted, the team can identify several different measures. For example, a team working to improve care for patients with myocardial infarctions may consider measuring pain management in the emergency room, the percentage of patients who receive beta-blockers, and the percentage of patients who receive coronary angioplasty with stenting of coronary vessels. They may also consider patient satisfaction, the number of days a patient misses work, the experience of the family of an acute myocardial infarction patient, or the number of patients who proceed to coronary artery bypass graft (CABG). These are all important considerations, but they cannot all be measured and monitored at the same time in a focused improvement project. Process modeling helps identify and prioritize the measures through the identification of key leverage points. (Chapter 6 describes the identification and linking of measures to a process.)

Process analysis helps generate hypotheses for change (Chapter 8). When a team starts its work to improve a system, many participants on the team think they know how to make the system better. These individuals may be on the right track, but a common model of the process helps to generate a greater number of possible approaches to improving the system. This process model helps a team see redundancy and waste in the system and figure out whether there are places to rearrange the steps or combine steps in the process. Similar to creating a list of possible diagnoses when a patient first presents for care, a process model is the key for generating a comprehensive list of possible changes.

Generating a process model is akin to creating a surgical plan for a patient. Surgery is much more than cutting, suturing, and tying knots. Successful surgery involves several steps, such as preparing the surgical site, assessing the patient's level of anesthesia, assessing the surgical site, accessing the anatomic location, and closing the surgical site. Each of these steps contains many subroutines that the surgical team performs. For example, because of the complex steps involved in a surgical procedure, it is vital that the care team understand both the anatomy and the physiology of the patient, each of which will affect the surgical approach. Similarly, process modeling identifies the anatomy of a system (in our case, a health care system). It determines the approach to improvement and makes improvement efforts more successful. Careful and thoughtful process modeling allows improvement team members to share their knowledge of a system of care, build a common understanding of how the system works, identify measures, and create a list of possible changes.

Culture, Context, and Systems

A process in health care is intimately related to the culture of a clinical setting, the context of clinical care, and the health care system.

Culture

Culture has been defined in many different ways. In a general sense, *culture* is used to denote a historically transmitted pattern of meanings and symbols by which people

Culture also refers to a pattern of learned, group-related perceptions—including both verbal and nonverbal language—that is added to values, the belief system, and the disbelief system.

communicate and develop their knowledge and attitudes about life.[1] This definition reflects the social aspect and development of culture. *Culture* also refers to a pattern of learned, group-related perceptions—including both verbal and nonverbal language—that is added to values, the belief system, and the *dis*belief system.[2] This definition is important because in it, culture tells you what is true and what is not true about the system in which you work. Students learn through this type of culture early in their clinical rotations, when more senior students pull them aside and tell them, "You learned quite a bit in your classroom work, but let me tell you how it *really* works around here."

Why does culture matter in a health care organization? Culture is a powerful, latent, and often unconscious set of forces that determines both individual and collective behavior. Culture has a strong influence on how both individuals and groups perform and behave. Cultural elements help determine the strategy and the modes of operation within an organization and should not be ignored. It is important to understand the role that culture plays in an organization when you set out to make the organization more efficient and effective.[3]

Culture is deep, broad, and stable, and it is an important feature of an organization. The depth of organizational culture provides direction and meaning to an individual's work. It provides tacit rules on how to do things. The breadth of organizational culture is a reflection of its expanse; thus, attempting to decipher culture can be challenging. Deciphering and understanding the culture of an organization takes time and provides explanations of why certain processes exist. One important feature of culture is that its stability makes it predictable. While the predictability of work routines is valuable, attempts to change culture often produce anxiety for everyone in the organization. The stability of culture also means that changing culture requires tackling some of the most stable (and possibly recalcitrant) parts of the organization.

A complimentary concept to culture in an organization is context of care.

Context

Culture is generally an accumulation over time of the actions, reactions, and artifacts within an organization. A complimentary concept to culture in an organization is *context of care*. *Context* refers to the circumstances in which a particular event or situation occurs.[4] *Context* derives from the Latin *contexere*, which means "to weave together." Just as context is important for understanding a story in literature, the context of clinical care processes provides a framework. Context is a local occurrence at a particular place and point in time that overlies the culture, which is the underlying and more stable part of the organization. One way to conceptualize this relationship is to think of the cross-weaving of context with an underlying culture.

In Figure 5-1 on page 61, elements of the context from the patient and family perspective interact and connect with elements of the context from the health care provider. These elements are interdependent, and they cannot easily be teased apart, nor do they need to be. Recognizing these elements provides information for describing, modeling, and understanding the context of care and the processes. Notice that some items are common to both sets of stakeholders: comfort with one another, financial issues, and previous health care experiences. The patient and family have factors related to the perception of illness, while health care workers may be affected by time pressures and competing demands (for example, other patients, research, teaching duties). The context and the underlying culture should not be ignored; identifying the particular elements in the context of care is an important part of improving care.

The complex interaction of culture and context. While identifying an organization's culture and context might seem simple on the surface, it quickly becomes quite complex. A health care system has many connections and interactions among its multitude of stakeholders: the patients and families, the nurses, the technology and information systems, the physicians, pharmacists, and the administrative staff. When we consider the different ways to view culture and context, these factors, and particularly the interactions between them, become numerous. The important point here is to appreciate the complexity and depth that culture and context play in the delivery of care; a specific culture and context are not inherently "good" or "bad" but

---

FIGURE 5-1. *Interwoven Elements of Context in a Clinical Care System*

Patient/Family Factors

Perception of illness · Previous health care · Financial issues · Family support · Comfort with system · Comfort with providers

Health Care Worker Factors

Time pressures
Competing demands
Previous care experiences
Payer expectations
Institutional support
Comfort with patient
Comfort with family

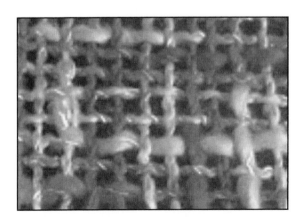

Source: Courtesy of Paul Batalden, M.D., and Leslie W. Hall, M.D. Printed with permission.

must be—and can be—recognized and described. Illustrating the processes, structures, and patterns of care is immensely helpful in making changes that are important, effective, and stable.

Systems

Culture and context exist within the different levels of a health care system. Identifying the levels of the system helps us to understand the context. A *system* is a set of interdependent elements working together to achieve a common aim. These elements may be both human and nonhuman (for example, technology, equipment, information).

Levels of systems. One model for representing the levels of systems in health care is shown in Figure 5-2 on page 63.[5] This target diagram shows five nested levels of health care systems. The model helps us address the question "What system is the unit of practice, intervention, and measurement that we are studying and improving?" This model of nested levels maintains the patient at the center—the appropriate focus for all improvement activities. As we move out from the center, we encounter the individual care providers and patient system, the familiar patient–clinician dyad. The microsystem is the next level and is important because it represents the transition from "one clinician to one patient" care to "many clinicians to many patients" care.[6] This is the first level of population patient care. Moving out from the microsystem is the mesosystem, which represents the connections between microsystems (such as the department of nursing or division of cardiology). The next level is the macrosystem, which is the hospital or health system. The outer circle in the model represents the community, market, and social policy systems. In the model, each level of the system can influence the patient's context of care at the center—some are proximal and some are more distant from the patient and family experience.

Let's take a closer look at each level:

- **Self-care system:** The self-care system is the patient, the information, and the information technology needed to take action to maintain health or increase the level of personal well-being. For example, a patient who has asthma will take medicines daily and will monitor environmental triggers that might make the asthma worse. Perhaps she will monitor peak expiratory flow rate (PEFR) each day to track the progress of her asthma.
- **Individual care provider and patient system:** If you ask a patient, "Where do you get your health care?" the patient may respond, "My doctor is Dr. Jones." This reflects the system level of the individual care provider's relationship to the patient and family as well as the aim of their interaction. The aim of this interaction is important and differs depending on the type of practice and training of the clinician.
- **Microsystems:** Microsystems are a unique part of the health care system. They comprise the people who come together to care for a defined population of patients and their families.[7] Microsystems are clinicians, clinical and administrative support persons, information, information technology, and a

FIGURE 5-2. *Model of Nested Levels of the Health Care System*

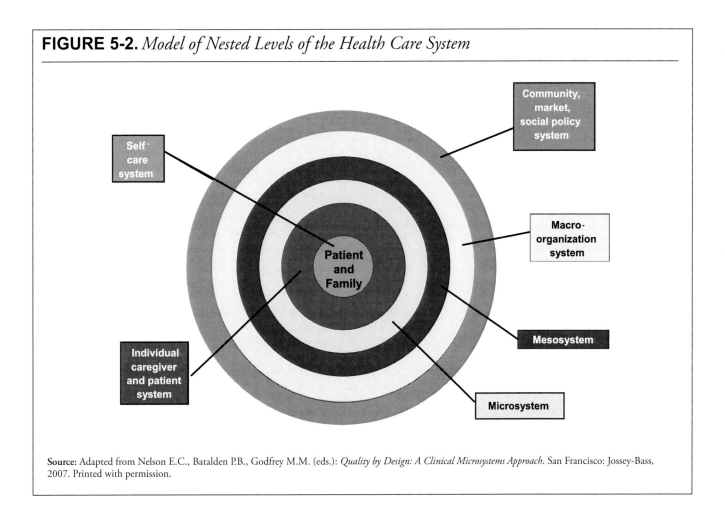

Source: Adapted from Nelson E.C., Batalden P.B., Godfrey M.M. (eds.): *Quality by Design: A Clinical Microsystems Approach.* San Francisco: Jossey-Bass, 2007. Printed with permission.

defined group of patients who come together for a specific health care purpose. The technology and information transferred between individuals is also part of the microsystem. The microsystem is a rich source of the context that influences the process on the front lines of care. The patients are a key part of the microsystem—not only on an individual basis but also on a population basis. The microsystem is the level at which you can start to identify and make changes for groups of patients.

■ **Mesosystem:** The mesosystem is the middle level of care delivery in an organization. It is the place where microsystems are linked and interact for patient care. This level often is identified by a service line (such as cardiac care center) or a department (such as medicine or nursing). Mesosystems often need to work together for a specific episode of care. For example, a patient with asthma who has an exacerbation presents to the urgent care clinic, requires admission to the intensive care unit for several days, and then completes her hospitalization on one of the medicine wards. Although she experienced care in three separate microsystems, her path through this episode was through the department of medicine mesosystem. However, systems at the same level can interact with one another. This patient could also be viewed as experiencing care in the department of nursing. This demonstrates the complexity of the systems approach to understanding care. The circles in our model do not depict the actual complexity of health care systems but provide a strong starting framework.

- **Macro-organization system:** A hospital, a clinic, or an integrated health care system or clinic that cares for a larger population is the macro-organization system. This can be either a single hospital or an integrated health network that cares for a group of patients across a region.
- **Society, community, market, and social policy system:** This is the geographic, political, and/or economic group of macro-organizations (for example, hospitals, payers, government) that have the aim of providing health care and fostering health in a community. For example, this part of the health care system encompasses the laws and environmental regulations that influence the health care of patients. It is unusual for these elements to directly influence individual patients, but they influence the policies and health care options that are offered through insurers, hospitals, microsystems, and individual providers.

Interactions among system levels. The model in Figure 5-2 is helpful in showing the different levels of the health care system, but how do these all fit together? Earlier, we mentioned a patient with asthma who monitors her PEFR at home. Let's suppose she has an office visit with her primary care provider every four months to review medications and symptoms (a patient–provider system). Between office visits, the patient has many interactions with the microsystem. She logs her PEFR values at a Web site that is reviewed regularly by a respiratory therapist affiliated with the provider's office. Also, the patient takes advantage of a home visit arranged through the local hospital (macro-organizational level). A nurse conducts the home visit to help the patient identify local environmental triggers for her asthma and to recommend changes to decrease the influence of the triggers. Although these health care workers are part of separate microsystems, they are under the mesosystems of the departments of medicine and nursing at the hospital. Finally, the patient is influenced by social policy and the health care market. She is a member of a health insurance plan that has changed the formulary recommendations for asthma medications, so she must switch brands of inhaled corticosteroids. This brief example shows that while the patient remains at the center of the health care system, her care may be affected by the many elements that occur at all levels of the system.

Culture, context, and systems are intimately linked to the processes of care. By understanding these elements, an improvement team can create a more reliable model of the processes of the care system. Input from all the team members helps to identify the cultural and contextual elements that influence efforts to improve care.

Process Modeling

Thus far in this chapter, we have discussed why understanding the culture, context, and system is important and how these concepts are related to one another. Next, we will explore a few of the methods that are available for creating process models.

Depending on the size and scope of an improvement project and the process to be understood, one or more methods may be needed. Becoming familiar with the methods discussed here (as well as other methods to model processes) provides a range of options to describe and understand processes of care. We present several of these tools, identify their strengths and limitations, and explore an example of each related to this chapter's opening vignette (*see* Table 5-1 below).

Brainstorming

While brainstorming might seem like a very simple technique, when it is appropriately facilitated, it can lead to a range of ideas that provide important insights into the processes of care. Table 5-2 on page 66, which shows the results of the opening vignette team's brainstorming session, demonstrates how this works. Having several people in the system of care involved in brainstorming helps the team identify aspects

TABLE 5-1.
Strengths and Limitations of Basic Process Modeling Techniques[8]

Modeling Technique	Strengths	Limitations
Brainstorming	• Enlists input from many individuals • Can be an important starting point • Generates a wide range of ideas and possibilities	• Brainstorming in a group must be facilitated • Must move beyond generating possibilities • Be wary of getting "stuck" on barriers
Cause-and-effect diagram	• Standard way to identify barriers in a system • Clearly identifies the end product of the system in the "head" • Stems and leaves identify specific aspects of the process	• No time aspect to the diagram (cross-sectional analysis tool) • Might be limited by the domains on the stems
Flow diagram	• Shows all parts of the process • Free flowing, so can represent all parts of the process • Standard symbols make interpretation easier • Can be annotated	• No clear link to individual or professional responsibilities • Can become cluttered by annotations
Deployment flowchart	• Same symbols as standard flow diagram • Shows people who perform each step • Columns for measures and change opportunities	• Challenging to fit on one sheet of paper • Often difficult to represent complex process with many stakeholders
Workflow diagram	• Uses a diagram of the physical layout to map the workflow pattern • Can show flow of people, information, or materials • Can often identify areas of duplication, waste, and handoffs in a process	• Challenging to show multiple patterns or variations in flow • Need accurate depiction of the physical layout of an area • Nonstandard processes might not show a consistent pattern

of the process that may have been hidden. For example, the front-desk check-in clerk on the improvement team described her challenges with the drop-in clinic. Although the drop-in system is also frustrating for the nurses and physicians, clinical staff are physically shielded from the waiting area. The front-desk clerks bear the brunt of patient inquiries. When patients become frustrated or angry with a long wait time, the front-desk clerks are left to manage the problems. The brainstorming session helped everyone involved to realize that this process encompasses more than just the clinical staff. The clinic support staff are key to the process as well. Any solutions for improvement will need to take this into account.

Cause-and-Effect Diagrams

A cause-and-effect diagram (also called an Ishikawa, or fishbone, diagram) is an excellent tool for uncovering and describing the range of factors that influence an outcome. There are three steps to creating this type of diagram:

1. A cause-and-effect diagram starts with the empty template (*see* Figure 5-3a on page 68). The box at the right side of the diagram contains a statement of the current problem to be solved. This is the effect, or the outcome, of the process being studied. This statement should be concise and to the point. This is not the same as the aim statement (Chapter 4) of the improvement team but just a clear statement of the specific problem. In Figure 5-3a, the statement is "Patients, staff, and clinicians are frustrated by long wait times in drop-in clinic."

2. The next step is to create headers (broad categories) for the stems on the diagram. Traditionally, six headers can be used: people, processes, policy,

---

TABLE 5-2.

Summary or Brainstorming Session by Drop-in Clinic Improvement Team (Nurse Practitioner, Physician, Front-Desk Clerk, Physician Assistant)

Discussion Question	Summary of Discussion
What works well at the current drop-in clinic?	• Each patient is seen on the day of his or her choice. • Not having to make appointments enables patients to simply show up at the clinic. • Other services in the hospital can refer patients to the clinic for evaluations. • Medical and nursing students get exposure to a range of urgent care conditions. • If the patient volume is low, the clinic's work may be completed early in the day.
What can be done better at the drop-in clinic?	• Although they do not have the information, front-desk clerks are often forced to field questions from patients about when they might be seen. • Patients do not know when they will be seen by a clinician. • Patient volume and acuity are difficult to anticipate. • If the patient volume is high, the clinic can run several hours over the limit. • Staff (clerks, nurses, clinicians) feel that they have very little control over the patient flow in the clinic.
How do we want to provide acute care for our patients?	• Our patients need access to acute medical care at our medical center. • The staff in the acute care area should have control over the flow in the clinic and be able to match available staff with patient volume.

methods, materials, and environmental factors (*see* Figure 5-3b on page 68). You may choose to use all or some of these, or you may choose to create labels that are appropriate for your team. (It is prudent to use at least three headers for a cause-and-effect diagram; using more than six headers often makes the diagram cluttered.)

3. The third step is to investigate each of the headers for more concrete examples. For example, under "people" in Figure 5-3c on page 69, you can see that the team entered the statement "Many new clinicians who are not familiar with the system," indicating that the group felt that the new clinicians were having difficulty with the clinic system. There are other examples under the other domains in Figure 5-3c.

This process continues around the entire diagram, with specific ideas placed on each of the bones. The cause-and-effect diagram is a hypothesis-generating tool, so any reasonable contribution should be added.

Flowcharts

A flowchart depicts the flow of a patient through a system, using a standard set of symbols. For example, Figure 5-4 on page 70 shows a flowchart for a patient in the drop-in clinic, the scenario presented at the beginning of this chapter. A flowchart is free flowing and can be annotated. The example in Figure 5-4 shows that a large portion of the patient's time is spent in the waiting room. This validates the results of the brainstorming session: When patients become frustrated about long wait times, the front-desk staff are the first who are approached with questions because they are the ones in close proximity to the patients in the waiting room. A standard flowchart is limited because there are no clear links to individual or professional responsibilities. Also, because it may contain many annotations, a flowchart can become quite cluttered and perhaps not easily interpreted.

Deployment Flowcharts

Another process modeling tool, a deployment flowchart (also called a swim-lane diagram), uses the same symbols as a standard flowchart and has the added benefit of identifying the individuals who interact with the patient at certain stages. A deployment flowchart includes columns for measures of each stage of the process and opportunities for improvement at each stage of the process. Figure 5-5 on page 71 represents the same process as in Figure 5-4. You will note in Figure 5-5 that even though the patient identifies his visit as being with the clinician, the majority of the patient's time is spent interacting with other individuals. This demonstrates the microsystem at work in the drop-in clinic. The change from a "no appointment necessary" to an "appointment only" clinic will affect all who work in this clinic.

Workflow Diagrams

A workflow diagram (also referred to as a transportation, or spaghetti, diagram) uses the physical layout of a setting to show the flow of people, materials, or information.

FIGURE 5-3. *Cause-and-Effect Diagrams of Possible Causes of Frustration with Long Wait Times in the Drop-in Clinic*

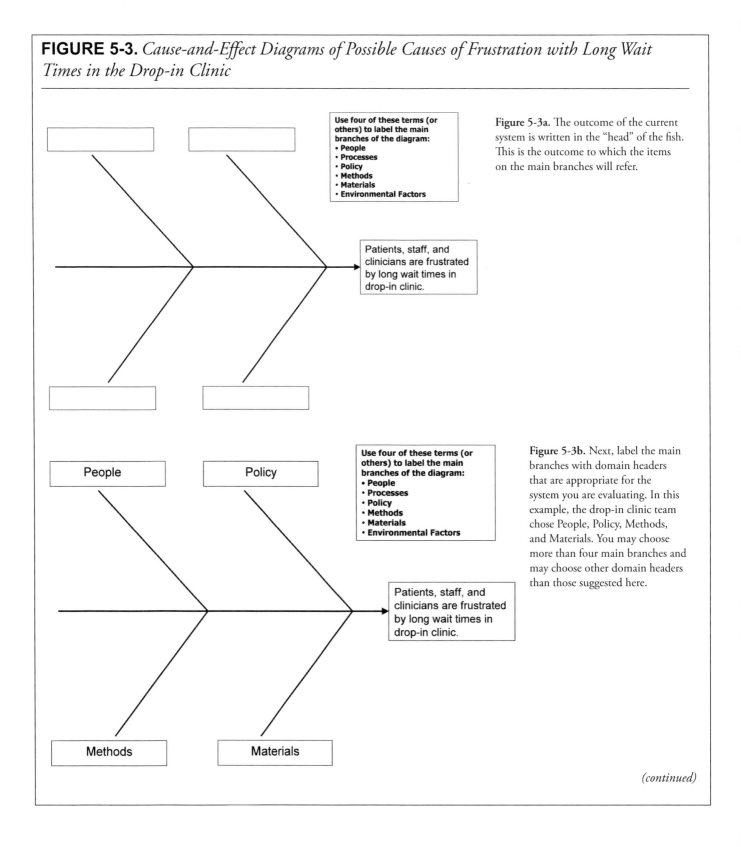

Use four of these terms (or others) to label the main branches of the diagram:
• People
• Processes
• Policy
• Methods
• Materials
• Environmental Factors

Patients, staff, and clinicians are frustrated by long wait times in drop-in clinic.

Figure 5-3a. The outcome of the current system is written in the "head" of the fish. This is the outcome to which the items on the main branches will refer.

People

Policy

Use four of these terms (or others) to label the main branches of the diagram:
• People
• Processes
• Policy
• Methods
• Materials
• Environmental Factors

Patients, staff, and clinicians are frustrated by long wait times in drop-in clinic.

Methods

Materials

Figure 5-3b. Next, label the main branches with domain headers that are appropriate for the system you are evaluating. In this example, the drop-in clinic team chose People, Policy, Methods, and Materials. You may choose more than four main branches and may choose other domain headers than those suggested here.

(continued)

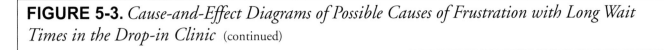

FIGURE 5-3. *Cause-and-Effect Diagrams of Possible Causes of Frustration with Long Wait Times in the Drop-in Clinic* (continued)

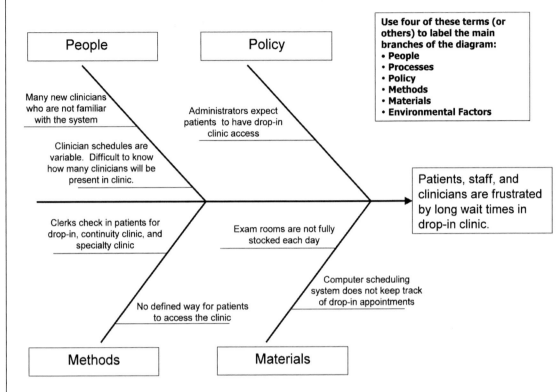

Use four of these terms (or others) to label the main branches of the diagram:
• **People**
• **Processes**
• **Policy**
• **Methods**
• **Materials**
• **Environmental Factors**

Figure 5-3c. Now add specific examples on the main branches. These are not to identify blame for the outcome but are to represent the range and depth of factors that contribute to the outcome.

This type of diagram is effective for showing waste in movement by individuals, showing delays in processing information, and identifying places where handoffs between individuals occur.[8] Figure 5-6 on page 72 shows a workflow diagram for one of the triage nurses in the drop-in clinic for the care of one patient. Notice how the nurse must travel from the triage room to the area by the front-desk clerk to retrieve paper from the printer, then to call the patient from the waiting room, and to another area to converse with the physician in the examination room and assist the patient to the procedure room. The movement of the nurse shows several areas of redundancy in which his actions could be more efficient. The workflow diagram provides a complementary process analysis to the other models when the goal is to create efficient and reliable flow in a system.

Notice how each process model (Figures 5-3, 5-4, 5-5, and 5-6) indicates that each patient spends a good deal of time waiting, but each depicts this slightly differently. There is no right or wrong process model; you can choose the one that best represents

There is no right or wrong process model; you can choose the one that best represents the system, context, and culture on which you are working.

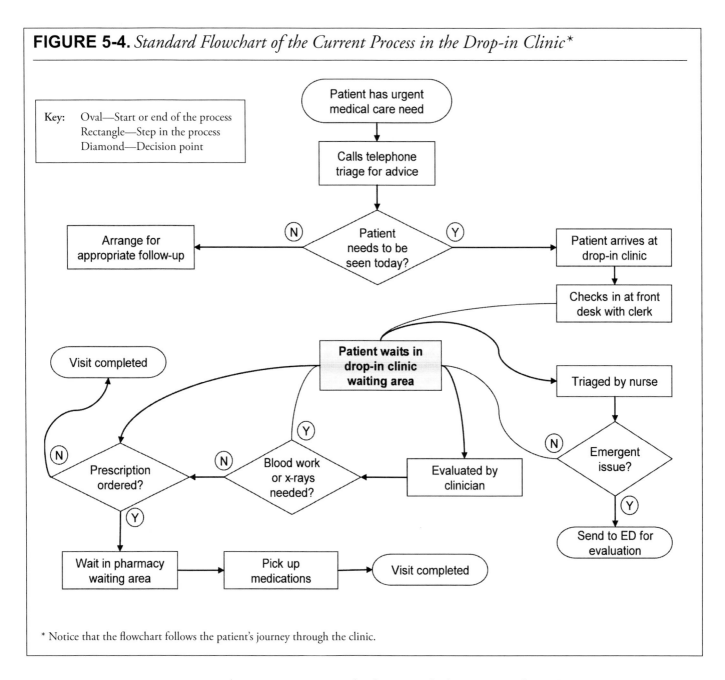

FIGURE 5-4. *Standard Flowchart of the Current Process in the Drop-in Clinic**

Key: Oval—Start or end of the process
Rectangle—Step in the process
Diamond—Decision point

* Notice that the flowchart follows the patient's journey through the clinic.

the system, context, and culture on which you are working. Sometimes, as in our example, you may even create several versions of the same process and choose the ones that are most helpful to your improvement team. With any process model, it is important to elicit feedback from everyone who is part of the process as part of the

FIGURE 5-5. *Deployment Flowchart of the Current Process in the Drop-in Clinic**

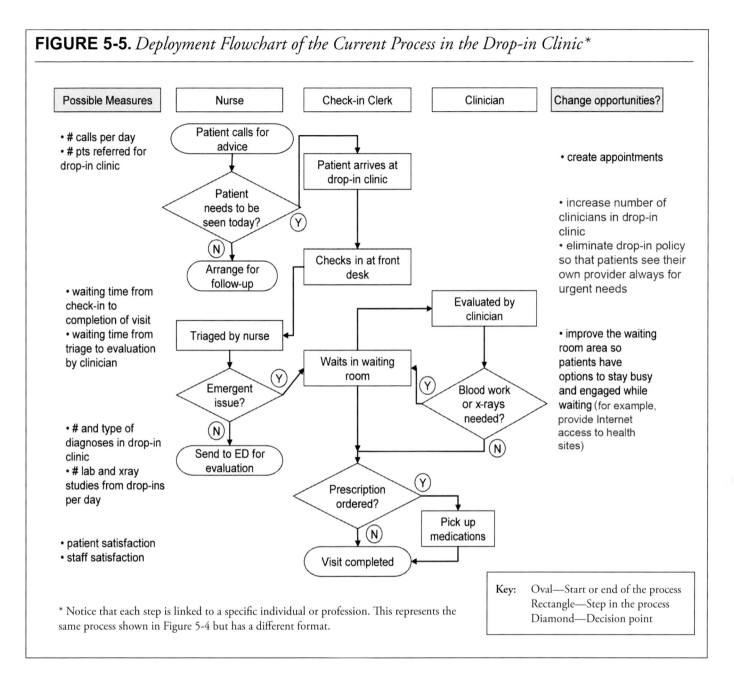

* Notice that each step is linked to a specific individual or profession. This represents the same process shown in Figure 5-4 but has a different format.

validation. Each process model that the team creates should be circulated to others who are part of the process, posted in a common area with an invitation to add comments, and ideally shared with patients and their families. This vetting step will improve the process model and focus the improvement on the patient experience.

FIGURE 5-6. *Workflow Diagram for One Nurse in the Drop-in Clinic for the Care of One Patient**

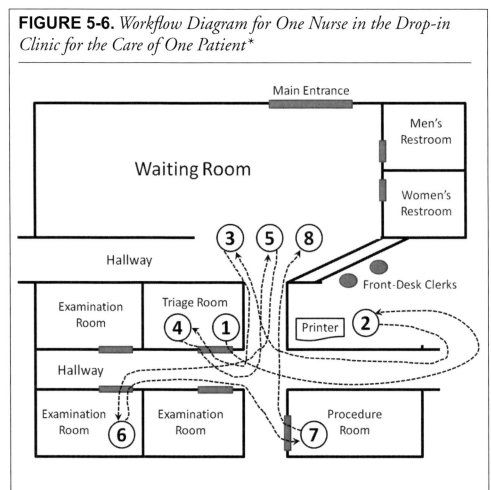

* Notice the high-traffic area in the main hallway and the multiple steps required for the movement of one patient through a drop-in clinic visit.

Summary

Process literacy is an important step in improving care. A common model of the care process is produced for the improvement team to discuss. In the Model for Improvement (*see* Figure 1-5 on page 10 in Chapter 1), a process model provides the necessary bridge between identifying measures and making changes. There are many tools available for process modeling. As with any other set of tools, practice and trial-and-error are key in helping to develop skills. You can practice developing and interpreting process models by mapping the processes around you: your morning routine, your study patterns, or a patient visit at a clinical site or hospital. Process modeling builds process literacy and provides insight into the many people, patterns, and structures involved in the delivery of care.

Study Questions

The following scenario describes a clinical care process in which a woman needed a stat C-section to deliver her baby. After you read the scenario, you will complete a fishbone diagram to determine some of the causes for the delay in the process. You will then create either a process flowchart or a deployment flowchart to depict what occurred. Finally, you will review the fishbone diagram and the process map to identify opportunities to improve this process.

Physician Magda Mooney is worried. She is driving to the hospital quickly, and her pager is ringing again. She knows that Emily LaFountaine presented to the labor and delivery ward ready to deliver. Her contractions are about 4 minutes apart, but her cervix is not expanding as quickly as would be expected. When Magda was called at home 10 minutes ago, it was obvious that the patient needed a C-section as soon as possible.

Magda arrives at the labor and delivery ward and is surprised to see that Emily is still in a delivery room. The charge nurse says that the hospital policy is to not move the patient to the operating room (OR) until the attending physician is present. Now Emily needs to be transferred to a gurney and transported to the OR. Oh, great—a delay. And where is the nurse anesthetist? He was supposed to arrive before the physician to place the spinal needle for anesthesia for the C-section. The labor and delivery clerk says that the call schedule had been changed at the last minute, so she had been paging the wrong on-call person. They figured out who was on call, and he is just arriving at the hospital. Another delay! At least Emily looks comfortable, and the baby's vital signs are looking okay, too.

Finally, the OR crew is assembled, and the patient is in the OR. The team performs a successful C-section, but the first incision occurred 52 minutes after the decision was made to go to C-section. National guidelines state that the decision-to-incision time should be less than 30 minutes. The patient and the baby are doing fine, but the frustration with the stat C-section process is evident to everyone. If only they could understand some of the issues that cause such variability in this process.

1. Complete the following fishbone (cause-and-effect) diagram. Start at the "head" of the fish, with a clear and concise statement of the problem. Then fill in the boxes with categories. Finally, add specific items to each of the main branches.
2. Create a process flowchart or a deployment flowchart of the current process in this scenario. Be clear about where the process starts and where it ends. You may add extra details that may not be apparent in the description of the case.

3. Generate a list of possible changes that may be tried to fix this problem. Use your fishbone diagram and flowchart to guide your decision making.

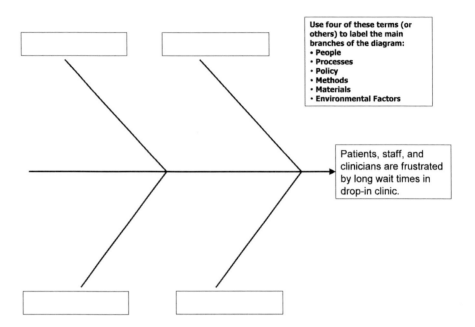

Use four of these terms (or others) to label the main branches of the diagram:
• People
• Processes
• Policy
• Methods
• Materials
• Environmental Factors

Patients, staff, and clinicians are frustrated by long wait times in drop-in clinic.

References

1. Geertz C.: *The Interpretation of Cultures*. New York: Basic Books, 1973.
2. Singer M.: *Intercultural Communication: A Perceptual Approach*. Upper Saddle River, NJ: Prentice-Hall, 1987.
3. Schein E.: *The Corporate Culture Survival Guide: Sense and Nonsense About Culture Change*. San Francisco: Jossey-Bass, 1999.
4. Morris W., ed.: *The American Heritage Dictionary of the English Language*. Boston: Houghton Mifflin, 1981.
5. Nelson E.C., Batalden P.B., Godfrey M.M. (eds.): *Quality by Design: A Clinical Microsystems Approach*. San Francisco: Jossey-Bass, 2007.
6. Batalden P.B., Ogrinc G., Batalden M.: From one to many. *J Interprof Care* 20:549–551, Oct. 2006.
7. Nelson E.C., et al.: Microsystems in health care: Part 1. Learning from high-performing front-line clinical units. *Jt Comm J Qual Improv* 28:472–493, Sep. 2002.
8. George M.L., et al.: *The Lean Six Sigma Pocket Toolbook: A Quick Reference Guide to 100 Tools for Improving Quality and Speed*. New York: McGraw-Hill, 2004.

CHAPTER 6

Measurement Part 1: Data Analysis for Improvement

OBJECTIVES

After reading this chapter, you will be able to do the following:

1. Explain why data are necessary for the improvement of health care.
2. Describe the differences between data used for research, for accountability, and for improvement.
3. Define the concept of a balanced set of measures for improvement work.
4. Describe one model—the clinical value compass—for identifying measures for improvement.

It's time for interprofessional rounds. Douglas Mandel, a surgical physician intern in his second month of residency training, Elizabeth Larsen, a nurse on the surgical floor with 8 years of experience, and the surgical team are all in attendance. Their first patient is Annette Quinn, a 73-year-old woman in postop day six for a partial colectomy for her persistent bleeding and symptoms of diverticulitis. As Douglas greets her with a "Good morning," he notices that she looks concerned. She tells the team, "My belly hurts a lot this morning . . . the incision seems to be burning. It felt much better yesterday." Elizabeth, the nurse, reports that the patient had a fever of 38.3°C (101°F) this morning and that the midline incision was reported as looking angry, red, and swollen. A small amount of pus was draining from the inferior part of the wound. After the team examines Annette, Douglas explains to her that it appears she has an infection and needs antibiotics.

The team finishes rounding on the other patients. Douglas approaches the attending physician, a general surgeon for more than 25 years who has a wealth of experience with patients, surgical technique, and complications. As they discuss Annette's wound infection, the attending listens to the story and comments, "That's always a risk with surgery. Be sure to stay sterile and carefully change the dressings postop."

Douglas, troubled by this reply, says, "I read an article about the appropriate timing of preoperative antibiotics. When I checked the chart, I saw that Mrs. Quinn's antibiotics were not started on time and that she received only one dose. The guidelines recommend that antibiotics be started before the incision and continued for 24 hours afterward.[1] It appears that Mrs. Quinn never received any antibiotics after the surgery. Do we know how often this occurs?" The attending ponders this question and replies, "I'm not a proponent of these types of guidelines. Guidelines might be helpful for some, but they often interfere with your decision making as a physician. It really is just 'cookbook medicine.' Wound infections are always a risk of surgery, particularly abdominal surgery." Douglas pushes back, "But perhaps this is an issue for other patients on the surgical service?"

At this time Elizabeth returns and says, "I was able to get some data about postop wound infection from our unit manager. We've had an 18% increase in postsurgical infections on the unit over the past eight months." The attending glances at the numbers and says, "Hmm . . . that's a cause for concern. Much higher than I would've guessed. Perhaps we should look into this in a little more detail." Elizabeth invites Douglas to be part of an improvement team to investigate and improve the timing of perioperative antibiotics. They make a plan to meet later that day to get started.

The Importance of Data for the Improvement of Health Care

Unfortunately, the attending physician's attitude in the above vignette is still too common. For many years, the public entrusted health care workers—particularly physicians—with providing good-quality care. This was seen as their professional duty and was assumed to occur based on the extensive education and training each had received. The public, and more specifically patients, believed that because clinicians gained knowledge and skills from school and clinical training, they were capable of providing reliable and high-quality care. Care was directed at each individual patient, and outcomes were determined by how each patient fared. Health care will always be directed to each individual patient, but over the past 25 years, there has been a shift to evaluating outcomes of groups of patients and providers. This shift in perspective is rooted in outcomes research and data evaluation; using data to evaluate outcomes is necessary for the improvement of health care.

Historical Foundations for Using Data to Improve Care

The foundation for using data to understand the outcomes of medical care and offer suggestions for improvement was seen as early as the mid-1800s. Central to this development were a young army nurse and a medical student.

Florence Nightingale's polar-area diagram. Florence Nightingale's work as a nurse for the British army is an excellent example of using data to improve care. During the Crimean War (1854–1856), she traveled with the army and cared for injured soldiers in the field hospital.[1] She was appalled to find that the mortality rate for soldiers in the field hospital was much higher than for soldiers at home. She recognized that while many soldiers were injured, the soldiers seemed to be dying more from complications of their wounds than from the wounds themselves. Within just six months of arriving at Scutari (located in what is now Istanbul), through improving sanitary conditions, she helped drop the mortality rate from 43% to 2%. Perhaps more impressive is that she devised a way to display the data and track the progress each month. Her polar-area diagram (also called a coxcomb chart) is a combination of stacked bar and pie charts that depicted the monthly number and causes of deaths (*see* Figure 6-1 below). Her presentation of data was so effective that it was shared with the *London Times* and with Parliament. Most importantly, her data display and analysis were the key to sharing the outcomes and the message with others, which led to interventions that greatly improved hospital sanitation and lowered mortality.

FIGURE 6-1. *Polar-Area Diagram of Preventable Deaths in British Soldiers per Month During the Crimean War, as Analyzed by Florence Nightingale*

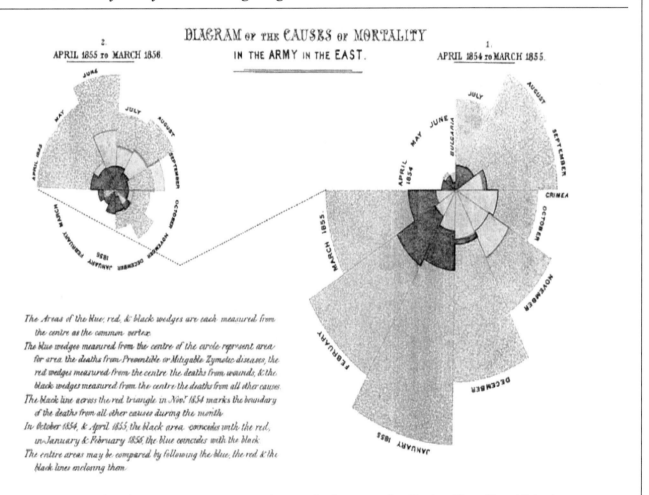

Source: Cohen I.B.: Florence Nightingale. *Sci Am* 250:128–137, Mar. 1984. Reprinted with permission from Houghton Library, Harvard University.

Ernest Codman's end-results system. In the late 1800s in Boston, Ernest Amory Codman was a medical student at Harvard.[2] During his surgery rotation, the medical students were responsible for administering anesthesia. One of his colleagues, Harvey Cushing, had a patient who became nauseated, vomited, and died as a result of this nausea and vomiting. The attending surgeon shrugged off the nausea and vomiting as "a usual part of anesthesia and surgery." Codman and Cushing were disappointed with this attitude and created a competition to see who could have the best patient outcomes in surgery. This competition led them to create anesthesia cards—some of the first medical records—that tracked the patient's name, operation, attending surgeon, and complications and included a graph of vital signs during the operation (*see* Figure 6-2 below).

Codman was passionate about the end results of patient care. The *end results system* was Codman's term for monitoring and assessing the outcomes of every patient encounter and creating a compendium of data for each patient until the end result was known. At a time when there was little, if any, record of patient progress or outcomes while in the hospital, Codman pushed for records of each and every patient encounter. He hoped to push health care from "art" to "science," but this was a notion whose time had not yet arrived. When he presented his system to colleagues and hospital leaders,

---

FIGURE 6-2. *Example of an Anesthesia "End Result" Used by Ernest Codman (c. 1910)**

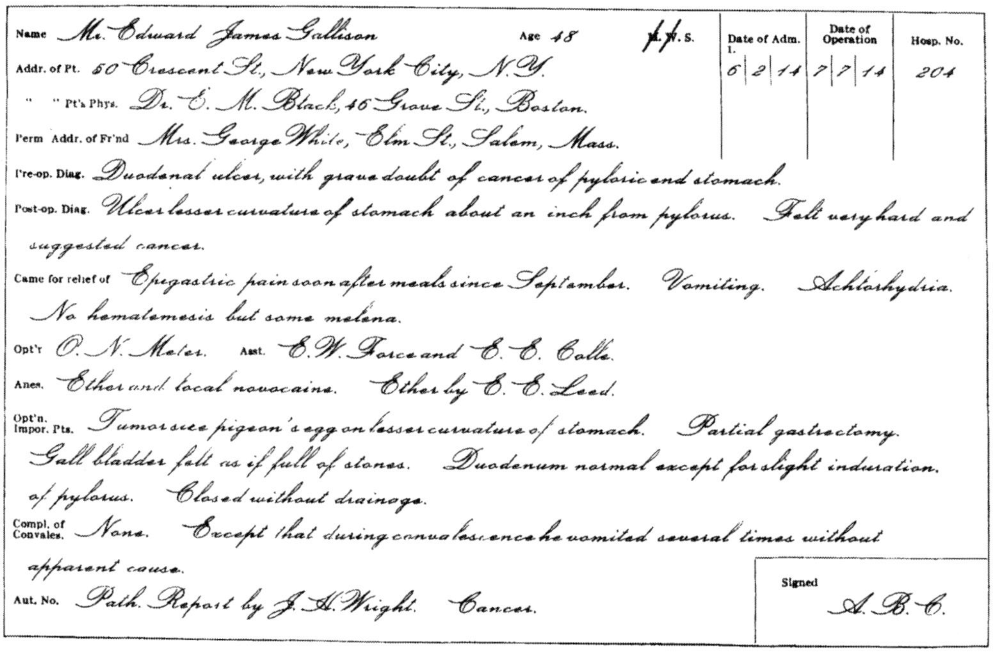

* Notice the simplicity of the information: patient name, age, gender, and medications administered.

Source: Donabedian A.: The end results of health care: Ernest Codman's contribution to quality assessment and beyond. *Milbank Q* 67(2):233–256, 1989. Copyright © 1989 Wiley-Blackwell Publishing. Printed with permission.

he was ostracized. His passion for the end result system resulted in a loss of income and stature in the medical community; however, his system was groundbreaking and was the foundation for medical records to establish accountability, monitor quality, advance clinical science, allocate resources, and even stimulate informed choices by patients and physicians.

Continued Struggles in Applying Data to Improve Care

Nightingale and Codman collected and analyzed data to understand the system of care. Their most significant contributions, however, were not the mere acts of collecting data and detecting patterns but rather that they were able to translate data into information for improvement. But why has their underlying message of analyzing and translating data into information for the purpose of system-level improvement not been readily and widely accepted within health care? Why is it still a struggle today to examine and use data in our clinical practices for improvement? Why are providers often reluctant to have anyone look at their data and results?

Building Measurement Knowledge

While the act of measuring health care processes and outcomes has increasingly become an integral part of the health care experience, most health care professionals (clinical as well as administrative) are not given sufficient grounding in measurement methods and statistical applications to cope adequately with the growing demands being placed on them to collect and analyze data for improvement. At some point, most health care professionals likely have learned about statistics, but overall there is relatively shallow knowledge in measurement principles and statistical methods, particularly those that are used in health care improvement.

There are many challenges along the measurement journey,[3] and it is not particularly an easy journey. Measurement can be time-consuming and can feel like added work. It can be challenging to make sure data are accurate and consistent. Often we feel there are too many indicators or not the appropriate indicators for the work we do. On top of this, measurement can feel threatening if it is used against you. If data are gathered and not used—particularly not used to inform decision making—then people become disillusioned with the measurement process. The best of intentions around measurement can frequently become muddled.

If data are gathered and not used—particularly not used to inform decision making—then people become disillusioned with the measurement process.

There are also some tremendous benefits of measurement for improvement of care. When done right, it can help you make decisions and make you feel more confident about your decisions. Measurement allows you to keep tabs on what is going on and thus sets the stage for improvement of systems. For discussions with clinical and management colleagues, it can provide a common frame of reference and help focus on what is important. Finally, measurement moves us away from anecdotes ($N = 1$) and one person's view to a more comprehensive view of the functioning of the system.

Measurement and the Scientific Method

All measurement efforts can be traced back to the fundamental principles of the scientific method.[4] Measurement is integral to the scientific method, but it is only one component of this inductive/deductive process. Figure 6-3 below shows the major steps in this scientific approach and groups these steps in terms of inductive and deductive processes.[5]

The inductive/deductive process. Note that when we begin an inquiry process and decide to start by collecting data (on the right-hand side of Figure 6-3), this is the start of our measurement journey on the inductive side of the scientific method (that is, the "specific" side to the "general" side). We first select and define measures (addressed at the end of this chapter) and then proceed to the collection of data believed to reflect the defined measures. The final step of this inductive phase is to analyze the data. Once we have statistical output, we enter the deductive phase of the scientific method ("general" to "specific"). In this case, we are going to interpret the output and ask ourselves if the data confirm or refute the theories we had when we started data collection in the first place. There are times, however, when the general theoretical concepts initiate the process and then we enter those on the inductive side of the diagram to obtain data and see if the data confirm or refute our theories. Measurement plays an important role in this circular process, but, as Nightingale and Codman both demonstrated, measurement must be used in a context of inquiry and action to improve the care processes.

> *Measurement must be used in a context of inquiry and action to improve the care processes.*

FIGURE 6-3. *The Components of the Scientific Method, Organized by Inductive and Deductive Thinking*

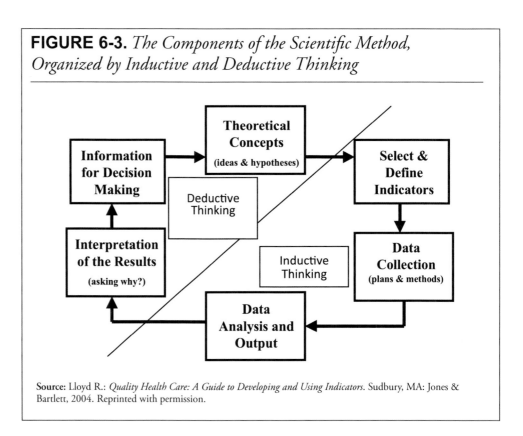

Source: Lloyd R.: *Quality Health Care: A Guide to Developing and Using Indicators.* Sudbury, MA: Jones & Bartlett, 2004. Reprinted with permission.

Fundamental Approaches to Measurement

All too often, health care professionals ignore the circular nature of the scientific method and view measurement of performance as if it were a singular event—and as if the same methods can be applied in all approaches to performance measurement. Nothing could be further from the truth. Solberg and his colleagues provide a strong starting point for thinking about different approaches to performance measurement.[6] They point out that there are three fundamental facets to performance measurement: improvement, accountability, and research. They explain the relationship among these three approaches to measurement as follows: "We are increasingly realizing not only how critical measurement is to the quality improvement we seek but also how counterproductive it can be to mix measurement for accountability or research with measurement for improvement."[6(p.135)]

The characteristics of each approach to measurement are shown in Table 6-1 below and are depicted in the rows. These aspects are basic requirements of any measurement approach. Each cell of this table describes how each aspect is applied for improvement, accountability, and research. Let's look at the columns individually to get a better understanding.

Research measurement. The basic aim of research is to develop new theories and knowledge or to test existing theories. Researchers ensure that designs control for exogenous variables that may create confounded results. Experimental designs are used to maximize the validity and reliability of the results. Researchers often collect more data than is needed in the event that reviewers, journal editors, or critics raise questions

---

TABLE 6-1.

The Characteristics of the Three Types of Measurement in Health Care

Aspect	Improvement	Accountability	Reasearch
Aim	Improvement of care	Comparison, choice, reassurance, spur for change	New knowledge
Methods **• Test Observability**	Test observable	No test, evaluate current performance	Test blinded or controlled
• Bias	Accept consistent bias	Measure and adjust to reduce bias	Design to eliminate bias
• Sample Size	"Just enough" data, small sequential samples	Obtain 100% of available, relevant data	"Just in case" data
• Flexibility of Hypothesis	Hypothesis flexible, changes as learning takes place	No hypothesis	Fixed hypothesis
• Testing Strategy	Sequential tests	No tests	One large test
• Determining if a change is an improvement	Run charts or Shewhart control charts	No change focus	Hypothesis, statistical tests (*t-test*, *F-test*, chi square) *p* values
• Confidentiality of the data	Data used only by those involved with improvement	Data available for public consumption and review	Research subjects' identities protected

Source: Solberg L.I., Mosser G., McDonald S.: The three faces of performance measurement: Improvement, accountability, and research. *Jt Comm J Qual Improv* 23:135–147, Mar. 1997.

about the results or methods.[6] Statistical analysis for research uses biostatistics, a branch of statistics that compares groups or that identifies the factors influencing the outcomes presented. The biostatistics in research measurement often produces a p value, which is helpful in interpreting the overall effect of the intervention as opposed to change from other factors. Measurement for research is an extremely important domain that essentially addresses the question of efficacy.[7] In everyday terms, research allows us to determine the efficacy of what is likely to work.

Accountability measurement. Measurement for accountability is used to compare and adjudicate outcomes of aggregate data. It is typically focused on making comparisons between groups and asking a very simple question: "Is performance better now that it was the last time? Yes or no?" In most instances, the answer is based on performance of the observed units against fixed targets or goals.

Improvement measurement. Finally, measurement for improvement is focused on monitoring the outcomes of a system over time to understand if the processes are efficient and effective.[8] It is intended to determine whether interventions have had significant effects on the performance and outcomes of a system. It is also focused on potentially how the processes relate to outcomes for patients. It is the extension of the research act. Traditional research helps us determine the "what," while improvement research allows us to determine the "how" (that is, how can we implement an efficacious idea, technique, procedure or drug so that it performs reliably every time it is administered or applied). A major distinction between improvement measurement and the other two types of measurement in Table 6-1 is that improvement incorporates statistical process control (SPC) methods (which we'll discuss in Chapter 7) to determine whether there has been a significant movement in the process performance. Statistical tests of significance (for example, p values) are not typically appropriate for improvement where analysis of the process variation over time is the determinant of improvement.

Navigating the Interfaces of Measurement Approaches

Health care organizations need leaders and frontline individuals who are comfortable and competent in being able to blend the three approaches to performance measurement. While some express that it can be counterproductive to mix the three approaches,[6] we do not view the three approaches as silos. Instead, we believe that it is more effective to view these not as independent and unrelated but rather as three facets of measurement. Health care leaders will improve their overall measurement capacity when they are able to navigate the interfaces of each measurement approach. Sometimes a person becomes strongly invested in only one approach to measurement. A person may talk about measurement for research as the "only" valid approach to measurement. Similarly, others may talk about aggregate and summary data that compare hospitals, cities, or regions. These individuals are invested solely in the measurement for accountability column. Institutions need individuals who can function as translators of these three approaches to measurement—who speak the language of each domain. For physician and nurse leaders, this is critical. They need to be able to walk comfortably back and forth across the columns in Table 6-1 so as to understand the valid, reliable, and solid measurement within each domain and not to be stuck in one measurement silo.

An example. An example will help to show how serving as a translator and moving between the three facets of performance measurement can be very beneficial. The *Dartmouth Atlas of Health Care* uses data from the U.S. Centers for Medicare & Medicaid Services (CMS), the health insurance program for individuals over age 65, to document local, regional, and national variation in outcomes and resources. The *Dartmouth Atlas* demonstrates geographic variation in aggregated outcomes and is used to compare performance between one locale or region and another. Table 6-2 below shows an example of comparison of aggregate data from the *Dartmouth Atlas* from 2007.[9] All scores are rather high, so with these data, it is difficult to determine any quality gap. These aggregated data at the state level can have an important utility for understanding accountability and differences between regions; however, aggregated data are of limited use for improvement within an individual hospital. Aggregated data presented in tabular formats or with summary statistics do not help you measure the impact of process improvements or redesign efforts. Aggregated data are useful not for improvement but for accountability.[5]

Aggregated data presented in tabular formats or with summary statistics do not help you measure the impact of process improvements or redesign efforts.

Understanding Variation in Measurement for Improvement

Because improvement of systems is the goal of our work in this book, we need to describe how measurement for improvement purposes differs from other types of measurement. What's missing? W. Edwards Deming was a U.S. physicist and statistician who worked in post–World War II Japan. He helped to rebuild Japanese industry after the war and has received much credit for the high quality of manufactured products in Japan. His work was translated to health care applications

---

TABLE 6-2.
Dartmouth Atlas Comparing Outcomes from Four States with a Composite Score and for Three Common Conditions*

State	Composite	Acute Myocardial Infarction	Chronic Heart Failure	Pneumonia
California	93	96	93	90
Connecticut	95	96	94	93
Massachusetts	94	96	93	92
New Hampshire	97	98	95	95

* Note that the score in each cell represents the technical process quality measure from 2007, 0 (low) to 100 (high).

Source: Adapted from Trustees of Dartmouth College: *The Dartmouth Atlas of Health Care.* http://www.dartmouthatlas.org (accessed May 5, 2011).

in the mid-1980s by Donald Berwick, M.D., Paul Batalden, M.D., and others, and it became the foundation for much of the modern quality improvement movement in health care. One of Deming's classic statements related to measurement and improvement was as follows: "If I had to reduce my message for management to just a few words, I'd say it all had to do with reducing variation."[10]

Understanding variation is vital to all improvement work. Let's take a practical example from the work of Carey and Lloyd[11] to show how recognizing the type of variation in data can help you take action on a system.

An example. Mary and Bill are both aiming shots at a target (*see* Figure 6-4 on page 85). Who is the better shot? Mary's shots are clustered together, but none hit the bull's eye. Bill's shots are more scattered, but he did hit the bull's eye once. A more appropriate question would be, "What does each person need to do to hit the bull's eye consistently?" It appears that Mary would merely need to adjust the sight of her rifle to the left and down slightly, while Bill would need to rethink his entire approach to shooting. His shots exhibit a random pattern on the target. If he continues with his current level of performance, how would he improve? If he adjusts his sight downward for his highest shot and gets it closer to the bull's eye, he will force the lowest shot on the target further away from the target. This example demonstrates why understanding the underlying variation in a system is so vital. If you are sincere and passionate about understanding where your processes have been, where they are now, and where they are headed in the future, then gaining knowledge about the type of variation and how to take action is key.

The impacts of not understanding variation. If you fail to account for the variation and understand its role, you can be tempted to misinterpret the data and overreact to individual data points. Lloyd outlines the impacts of not understanding variation[5]:

- You will be tempted to see trends where there are no trends.
- You will try to explain natural variation as special events.
- You will blame and give credit to people for things over which they have little or no control.
- You will have a distorted understanding of the process that produced the data.

Unfortunately, in health care, we demonstrate these behaviors on a regular basis. For example, it is not uncommon when reviewing data to state, "These data are not reliable or accurate for my organization. Our patients are different and have more serious health problems than those in other organizations." We are very good at denying the data, distorting the process that produced the data, or blaming the individual or organization that delivers the message. We do this by claiming that our patients are sicker, older, or more complex, or that the time has lagged so much that the data are not relevant anymore. Sometimes, this response is grounded in the belief that others should not be reviewing performance. At other times, it is because we know that the

FIGURE 6-4. *Example of Understanding Variation Within a Set of Data**

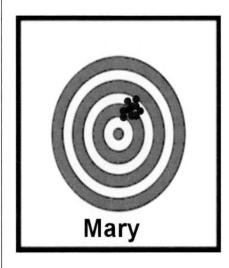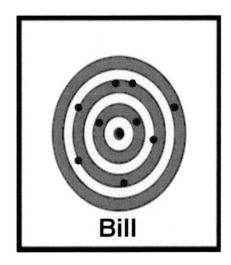

* Note that the data here are the individual shots on a target by each person. Each person takes 10 shots at the target.

Source: Reproduced by permission of Raymond G. Carey, Ph.D., and Robert C. Lloyd, Ph.D., *Measuring Quality Improvement in Healthcare: A Guide to Statistical Process Control Applications.* Milwaukee: ASQ Quality Press, 2001. To order this book, visit ASQ at http://www.asq.org/quality-press.

results are either not particularly good or the variation is considerable. Finally, it may be due to the fact that we have no idea what the variation is that lives in our data. Regardless of the motivating factors, without a clear understanding of the variation in our processes and outcomes, it is very difficult to provide reliable results or improve.

What improvement measurement should be. In summary, measurement for improvement guides us in how to take action on systems. This is distinctive and complementary to measurement used for research or accountability. Improvement measurement should be characterized by comprehensive, balanced data collection and analysis. It should be aimed at evaluating local systems and for knowing whether the changes that were made led to improvements. Measurement for improvement seeks to understand the outcomes in relation to the specific causal processes (that is, the context of care in a health care setting). Simply stated, measurement for improvement provides a basis for decision making. In Chapter 7, we will delve into the types of variation, how to use analytic tools to analyze variation, and how to link measurement to improvement strategies.

Sidebar 6-1. *Experiential Learning*

When you use data for improvement and to make decisions, you engage in a common cycle of experiencing and learning. David Kolb's[12] (1984) experiential learning cycle describes this process in more detail (*see* Figure 6-5 below). This is a process in which we engage each time we care for an individual patient and also when we focus on the system. We start, at the top of Figure 6-5, with a concrete experience. Recall that in this chapter's opening vignette, one of the team's patients had an unanticipated wound infection. Douglas Mandel, the surgical intern, reflected upon what this one case could mean in terms of the overall care of surgical patients. This is what we see in the right-hand part of Kolb's diagram. Douglas made an abstract generalization when he asked whether wound infections were a common occurrence at Parkside Hospital. The attending physician dismissed his question, saying that wound infections are "part of the usual course of practice."

FIGURE 6-5. *David Kolb's Experiential Learning Cycle**

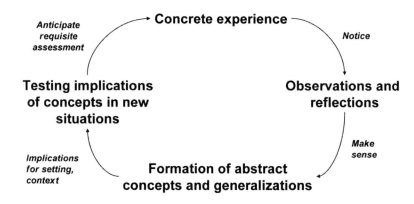

* "Testing implications of concepts in new situations" is the key step leading back to concrete experiences. Analytic data evaluation is an important part of this when applying Kolb's cycle to learning about systems. The level of data collection must align with the level of the system that is being considered.

Source: Kolb D.: *Experiential Learning: Experience as the Source of Learning and Development.* Upper Saddle River, NJ: Prentice-Hall, 1984. Copyright © 1984, page 25. Reprinted with permission of Pearson Education, Inc., Upper Saddle River, NJ.

This is where we get to the left-hand side of Kolb's model. Elizabeth Larsen, the nurse on the team, was ready to start testing the implications of a wound infection and whether the timing and duration of preoperative antibiotics was occurring in a reliable fashion. She helped to further explore this hypothesis by obtaining outcome data about wound infection on the ward. This combination of the data and the hypothesis led to the initiation of an interprofessional team with Elizabeth, Douglas, another surgery resident, a medical and nursing student, an operating room nurse, and a clinical pharmacist to identify the processes involved for perioperative antibiotic delivery. Initially, the utility of data for patient care was disregarded by the attending physician. Our patient, Annette Quinn, will likely recover from her infection and return home; however, the increased hospital stay, pain, and costs were unnecessary and could be avoided in the future if the system can learn from its outcomes and processes.

Kolb's model provides an opportunity to take our individual reflections and learn from them by forming concepts and generalizations and then retesting them through new situations. This cycle of learning is core to improvement work. Analysis of data plays a vital role of assessing and testing our generalizations and understanding whether generalizations are confirmed across many patient encounters. Understanding the variation in the data allows us to formalize the observation phase of Kolb's learning cycle at the system level.

Identifying a Balanced Set of Measures for Improvement

Inez Anton is a family physician who recently received a summary of data about her clinic's patients with diabetes. The report card is dreadful: The rate of yearly eye exams is low, hemoglobin A1c levels are higher than last year, and blood pressure control looks poor. The report card is an extraction of data from the charts and lab tests. It is summarized in a table with comparisons to "exemplary performers" in the region. Over lunch one day, she expresses her frustration at these outcomes and shares the report with Tomas Vucic, the practice administrator, and Marla Edissen, the senior nurse in the clinic. Inez comments that this is ridiculous, saying that the report card compares clinics that are not similar. She says, "This 'report card' is exasperating. . . . Who chooses these measures? I recognize our practice can get a bonus payment for good performance, but who makes these measurement decisions?"

Tomas and Marla look at the report and are just as perplexed. Marla states that their patients seem very satisfied with their care: "We get very few, if any, patient complaints." Tomas comments that the electronic medical record that started three months ago can provide trending data and analysis. He hasn't had the time to do this, and the information technology support group from the hospital has been too busy putting out fires in the new system to perform any data extraction. Once again, here is a system with lots of promise but little to show for it.

Together these three agree that there must be a nugget of reality buried in these report cards, but they are unsure how to study their local processes to improve care for their patients with diabetes. Marla and Tomas agree to take the next step and brainstorm about some ways the team can improve the delivery of care.

Before you can display and interpret your data (and understand the variation in it), you must identify appropriate measures for the system. Consider the famous quote "Some are born into leadership; others have it thrust upon them." It is similar with measures in health care: As we noticed in the vignette, sometimes measures are thrust upon us. A hospital or a health plan (or an insurance company) may recommend (or require) that a practice start measuring certain outcomes of care. A health plan may even "score" a practice based on these measures. Examples of these measures might include readmittance rate to a hospital for patients with congestive heart failure, adequate blood pressure control for patients with diabetes, or rates of immunizations. These measures are recommended—in fact, demanded—by external forces. This is the reality of health care systems, and it can sometimes be a reasonable point from which to initiate improvement; however, these measures of accountability are often not enough to support meaningful improvement.

The opportunity to identify your own measures may be daunting but provides a chance to define specific—and balanced—measures that are helpful to your team. Usually, a set of balanced measures may include data that are provided to you and data that you obtain on your own.

Using a Clinical Value Compass to Identify Measures

One helpful tool for identifying a complement of measures is the clinical value compass.[13] We'll discuss the concept of measuring the *value* of care and provide an example to show how the clinical value compass can be used to identify measures.

The value equation. In short, value is equal to quality divided by cost (that is, Value = Quality / Cost). This value equation comes into play whether you are buying a toaster, choosing a computer, or deciding which surgical group you will choose to do your hip replacement surgery. The clinical value compass (*see* Figure 6-6 on page 89) takes the value equation and divides quality into three domains: clinical, functional, and satisfaction. Costs are located at the southern point of the compass (as in the denominator of the value equation).

The value compass as a brainstorming tool. The clinical value compass is a brainstorming tool for identifying measures. (*See* Chapter 5, pages 65–66, for more information on brainstorming.) A team uses it by drawing an empty value compass on a sheet of paper, a whiteboard, or a flip chart. The team then "walks" around the compass—that is, the team brainstorms measures prompted by the points on the compass—and generates ideas. Some proposed measures might not fit exactly on one location. This is okay. It is best to get the ideas on the board so that a comprehensive set of measures can be identified. The measures will be edited in the next step.

The organization of the value compass. Figure 6-7 on page 90 is a value compass that a team is working on to identify measures related to improving care for patients with diabetes at a clinic, as in the vignette. Notice the aim statement at the top of Figure 6-7. As discussed in Chapter 4, the aim statement keeps the improvement effort focused. Also, note that the measures are from different perspectives and different stakeholders: patients, family, and staff. The "western" point of the compass (clinical) includes several measures, including average hemoglobin A1C, blood pressure control, eye exams, foot exams, and lipid control. At the functional ("north") point of the compass are measures related to patient hypoglycemic episodes and the number of patients enrolled in exercise programs. The satisfaction point ("east") contains elements of patient and family satisfaction with the office staff, the clinician, and the hospital. Also at this point is staff satisfaction with care for patients with diabetes. The southern point of the compass contains the costs, both direct and indirect. Direct costs are those that involve financial outlays such as medication expenses, hospitalization payments, and clinic payments. Indirect costs include days lost from work due to complications of diabetes.

The measures in Figure 6-7 are a combination of process and outcome measures. *Process measures* are those that evaluate actions that are directed to or known to influence the end result. For example, the percentage of patients who receive a foot exam is a process measure. Foot exams are not an outcome of diabetes but are an important process put in place to screen patients with diabetes for potential

---

DEFINED:
Process Measures

Process measures are those that evaluate actions that are directed to or known to influence the end result.

FIGURE 6-6. *Clinical Value Compass for Identifying Measures (Value = Quality / Cost)*

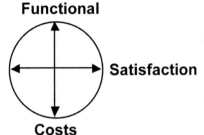

- Physical function
- Mental health assessment
- Social/role function
- Measures of health status (pain, vitality, perceived well-being)

Functional

- Mortality and morbidity
- Signs, symptoms
- Complications
- Diagnostic test results

Clinical   **Satisfaction**

- Patient, family, and caregiver satisfaction with health care delivery process
- Patient's perceived health benefits

Costs

- Direct medical costs (copay, hospital services, medications)
- Indirect social costs (time lost from work, caregiver costs)

Source: Nelson E.C., Batalden P.B., Lazar J.S. (eds.): *Practice-Based Learning and Improvement: A Clinical Improvement Action Guide*, 2nd ed. Oak Brook, IL: Joint Commission Resources, 2007.

---

lesions on their feet. An *outcome measure* is the end result of a process. Outcome measures are often the most important measures to measure because they represent the consequences of the processes. In this example, an outcome measure might be the number of patients who require foot amputation because of diabetes-related complications. It is the main outcome of interest, but it is too far downstream to be the only measure that is used. A combination of process and outcome measures is another component of balanced measures for improvement.

Choosing from possible measures. The list of measures in Figure 6-7 is extensive, and it will not be possible for the team to measure and evaluate *all* of these items; that would be impractical. The value compass helps identify *possible* measures. The team next needs to choose the measures it will use. Figure 6-7 also shows how the team narrowed the choices (circled items). Because percentage of patients with the hemoglobin A1C less than 7 and systolic blood pressure less than 130 have a strong correlation with clinical outcomes, the team chooses to focus on these at the clinical point on the compass. The functional measure will be the number of patient days with hypoglycemic (low blood sugar) episodes. The number of days with low blood sugar will need to be extracted from charts, but the team felt that this could be a reasonable and important proxy for a patient's participation in work and leisure activities. The

DEFINED:
Outcome Measures
Outcome measures are often the most important measures to measure because they represent the consequences of the processes.

A combination of process and outcome measures is another component of balanced measures for improvement.

FIGURE 6-7. *Clinical Value Compass for Improvement Team Working on Improving Care for Patients with Diabetes* *

Aim: Over the next nine months, we will increase the control of blood glucose and blood pressure by 50% for our patients with diabetes mellitus while keeping the costs for our patients unchanged.

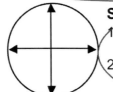

Clinical
1. Total # of patients with DM
2. Average HbA1C for all patients
3. % patients with HbA1C < 7%
4. % patients with systolic blood pressure < 130
5. % patients with foot exam
6. % patients with diabetic eye exam
7. # emergency department visits for diabetes related concerns
8. % patients with low density lipoprotein less than 100

Functional
1. # patients enrolled in exercise program
2. Total # hypoglycemic episodes per month

Satisfaction
1. Patient satisfaction with provider, office staff, and hospital
2. Staff satisfaction with care for patients with diabetes

Costs
1. Prescription medication costs
2. # office visits per month
3. Hospital charges
4. Days missed at work related to diabetes complications

* Circled items are the measures the improvement team decided to use for its project. See the text for a full description.

team also chose to focus on patient *and* staff satisfaction to gauge both sides of the clinical encounter. The team would like to measure days missed at work related to diabetes, but these data were too challenging to obtain. The team settled on the total number of office visits and average prescription medication changes for patients related to diabetes.

As you see in Figure 6-7, the team completes the value compass with a few measures at each point of the compass. This provides an array of measures to monitor care for patients with diabetes in the clinic. This collection of measures may not be perfect, but it is considered a good place to start. The group may drop or add other measures as its work on diabetes care continues.

Moving to operational definitions. The next step is to write an operational definition for each of the measures (*see* Table 6-3 on page 92). An *operational definition* is a specific, detailed description of the measure so that everyone on the improvement team and outside the team knows exactly what each measure describes. The operational definition might also include where the data are generated and gathered (such as lab test and chart review), who is responsible for obtaining the data (for example, office staff, insurance plan, an outside firm), and what is to be included in a numerator or denominator. While writing these definitions may seem laborious, the clarity the

---

DEFINED:
Operational Definition

An operational definition is a specific, detailed description of the measure so that everyone on the improvement team and outside the team knows exactly what each measure describes.

definitions provide will be well worth the effort as the project progresses.

Using the value compass to clarify measures: Qualitative or quantitative? When it is time to collect data for your measures, it is important to be clear about whether you are building qualitative or quantitative measures. This is a real strength of the value compass approach. For example, staff satisfaction could be assessed with a lunchtime feedback session, similar to a "focus group" approach. In this case, a qualitative evaluation through structured discussion will provide greater depth of responses than a quantitative survey. This could be a convenient and nonthreatening opportunity for some directed feedback about diabetes care. At other times, we deal with more quantitative data. For example, data that are gathered and reported quarterly by an insurance company or government agency are typically quantitative in nature and consist of counts, percentages, rates, or scores. The time interval or frequency of each assessment is also important to consider. Values such as percentage of patients with systolic blood pressure less than 130 and percentage of patients with HbA1c less than 7.0% could be extracted monthly from the electronic medical record (with assistance from the information technology staff). This would allow a quicker turnaround time for identifying whether a change in the care process makes a difference in the outcomes.

Using Other Data Instruments or Collection Methods

Other data may require new instruments or collection methods. Although the practice in our vignette reports no patient complaints, how much does the team know about the overall satisfaction from their patients with diabetes? The team may want to use a standardized survey that is sent to diabetic patients (or to all of the team's patients) to assess their satisfaction. This would allow the team to then make changes that directly attend to patient needs. Perhaps the office staff would focus on more than the office microsystem or the patient–preceptor dyad and find ways to help patients in their personal care system. (*See* the discussion in Chapter 5 regarding context and systems.) In Table 6-3, notice that the team does not have a way to assess patient satisfaction, so it is planning to enlist an outside agency to help survey its patients.

No one piece of data provides the entire story of the clinical system under investigation, and not one of these measures is more important than another. Because the systems in which we work (and where patients receive care) are complex, a balanced set of measures can account for clinical outcomes, patient functional and satisfaction status, and costs. These measures—identified with the value compass— help you assess the system and make decisions for improving many aspects of care.

Displaying Measures for Analysis

Once measures are chosen, it may be cumbersome to follow multiple measures in several electronic files or on many sheets of paper. Although it may not be possible for every improvement project, bringing together the measures into a comprehensive display as a data dashboard can be very helpful.[14]

TABLE 6-3.

Operational Definitions for the Measures Identified in Figure 6-7

Measure	Operational Definition
Total # of patients with DM	Number of patients in our practice who carry diagnosis of diabetes mellitus (DM), type 1 or type 2
% patients with HgbA1c<7%	Of those patients with DM who have had an HgbA1c drawn in the past 12 months, what percentage (or proportion) have a value less than 7?
% patients with systolic blood pressure <130	Of those patients with DM, what percentage (or proportion) of patient's most recently recorded systolic blood pressure is less than or equal to 130?
# hypoglycemic episodes per month	The total number of low blood sugar reactions reported by all of our patients
Patient satisfaction	To be determined once we find a suitable satisfaction survey for our patients
Staff satisfaction	Major themes of DM care from the perspective of all members of our staff
Prescription costs	Total costs (not just copay) incurred each month for DM–related medications and supplies
# office visits per month	Total number of office visits per month that are coded for 250.XX (diabetes-related care)

Data Dashboards

A data dashboard is sometimes confused with a report card. While a report card conjures up visions of judgment on a specific task (pass/fail), a dashboard is intended to monitor and provide feedback on the state of the system, whether it's a car traveling along the highway or an office providing care to diabetics (as in our example). Figure 6-8 on page 93 is an example of a dashboard for diabetes care. In the center, you see the value compass, which is always present to orient the data. At the clinical point, notice that the data about the number of patients with diabetes and the two outcome measures we chose to focus on are displayed in graphs. These are statistical process control charts, or more simply "control charts." Using these charts is one way to assess the variation in data. We will cover these charts in detail in Chapter 7. For now, just recognize that each data point is a summary of monthly data, and each month when the data are extracted, another point is added to each chart.

The functional point of the compass also has a control chart. However, since the team needed to gather the information about the number of low blood sugars per month, there are only a few data points on this chart. Each month, another data point will be added to the chart, so the information will grow as the data grows. The satisfaction point contains a summary of the staff feedback about diabetes care and a note that patient satisfaction surveys have been received from three companies. The practice will need to decide which survey to use. Finally, the cost data are also noted in control charts. The prescription cost is broken down by types of medicines, and the number of office visits per month for diabetes is summarized from the electronic medical record.

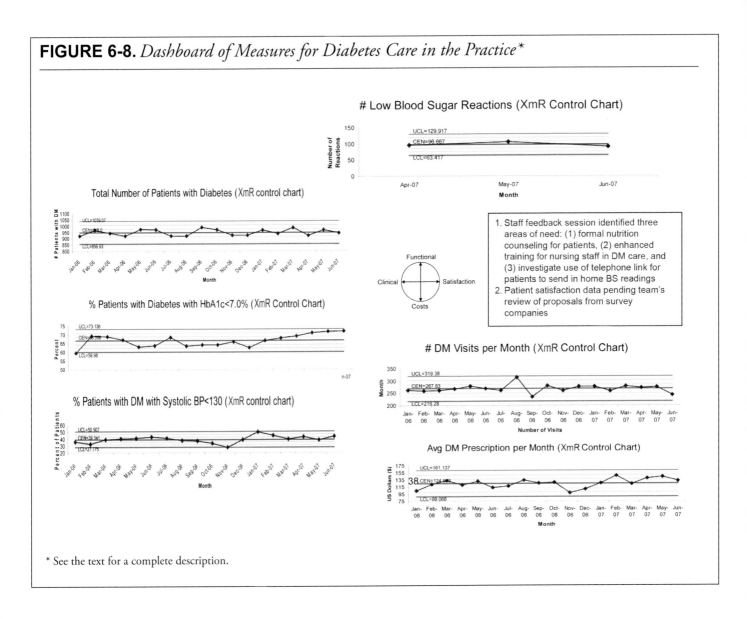

FIGURE 6-8. *Dashboard of Measures for Diabetes Care in the Practice**

* See the text for a complete description.

This dashboard allows for a quick overall assessment of the various measures for the office system. For example, perhaps the team recommends to start prescribing a new, rather expensive diabetes medication in hopes of increasing the percentage of patients whose hemoglobin A1c is < 7.0%. If the prescriptions costs start to rise, with no concomitant increase in the percentage of patients under control, the team will be able to recognize this as the data are charted. This demonstrates one of the benefits of using multidimensional, balanced measures.

Summary

Measurement alone is not sufficient for improvement, but it is one of the key steps in the model for improvement. Aggregate data in tabular format is best used for accountability and often leads to judgment, not improvement. While summary data for accountability has a role in the comparison of systems, regions, or countries, it is limited in its utility for improvement. Thoughtful analytic studies focus on gaining insight into the system that produces outcomes and are an essential component of improvement.

Data analysis for improvement starts with identifying measures. The clinical value compass is one tool that can help a team identify balanced measures for a project. By focusing on the *value* of care delivered, the team can address both the quality and costs within the system. Although often there are more data and more measures than a team can reasonably handle, the team chooses which measures to use that will give the best overall assessment of the system the team is trying to improve.

Study Questions

A medical student and a nurse practitioner student are paired to work in a hemodialysis unit. Hemodialysis *is the process of extracting fluid and solutes from the serum of patients with severe acute and chronic renal failure. Patients with chronic renal failure who require hemodialysis come to the unit three times per week to be dialyzed for three to four hours each time. At the end of the first week, the dialysis nurse manager invites the students to join in their hemodialysis quality improvement (HDQI) meeting.*

In preparation for the meeting, the manager suggests that both students begin to pay attention to the processes and flow in the unit. The students notice that patients arrive and are generally in good spirits each morning. By midday and into the afternoon, the mood on the unit changes considerably. Patients and family members are frustrated and angry that the hemodialysis times are running late. They state that they need to get back to work, and the time overruns are very inconvenient. The students talk with several patients who were scheduled for a three-hour dialysis run but are now close to four hours. One patient says he had just been in the hospital for a bloodstream infection that he suspects he got from the hemodialysis center. Another patient relates that she has a temporary dialysis catheter because her arterial-venous graft was not mature enough when dialysis needed to start. The students can see that there are many opportunities for improvement in this unit.

At the HDQI meeting, the topic for the day is measurement. Much of the discussion focuses on the number of dialysis slots, how many patients are being served, and the recent financial statement. The nurse manager expresses his frustration at these one-dimensional data and puts a value compass on the whiteboard to expand the conversation about measures.

1. Use the scenario above (and other information you may have about hemodialysis) to create a set of possible measures for the hemodialysis unit. The value compass is intended to make you think broadly: It is a brainstorming tool, so be creative for each point on the compass. Also, consider many perspectives (for example, patient, family, clinicians) when creating measures.

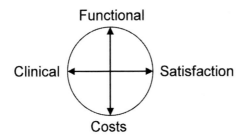

2. Write an operational definition for one measure from each point in your value compass. An operational definition is a specific and detailed description of the measure so that everyone recognizes exactly what each measure describes. It might include where the data are generated and gathered (such as a lab test or a chart review) and who is responsible for obtaining the data (for example, office staff, insurance plan, an outside firm).

Measure	Operational Definition
Clinical	
Functional	
Satisfaction	
Costs	

References

1. Cohen, I.B.: Florence Nightingale. *Sci Am* 250:128–137, Mar. 1984.
2. Donabedian A.: The end results of health care: Ernest Codman's contribution to quality assessment and beyond. *Milbank Q* 67(2):233–256, 1989; discussion 67(2):257–267, 1989.
3. Lloyd, R.: Navigating in the turbulent sea of data: The quality measurement journey. *Clin Perinatol* 37:101–122, Mar. 2010.
4. Lastrucci C.: *The Scientific Approach: Basic Principles of the Scientific Method.* Rochester, VT: Schenkman, 1967.
5. Lloyd R.: *Quality Health Care: A Guide to Developing and Using Indicators.* Sudbury, MA: Jones & Bartlett, 2004.
6. Solberg L.I., Mosser G., McDonald S.: The three faces of performance measurement: Improvement, accountability, and research. *Jt Comm J Qual Improv* 23(3):135–147, Mar. 1997.
7. Glasziou P., Ogrinc G., Goodman S.: Can evidence-based medicine and clinical quality improvement learn from each other? *BMJ Qual Saf* 20(suppl. 1):i13–i17, Apr. 2011.
8. Carey, R.G.: *Improving Health Care with Control Charts: Basic and Advanced SPC Methods and Case Studies.* Milwaukee: ASQ Press, 2003.
9. Trustees of Dartmouth College: *The Dartmouth Atlas of Health Care.* http://www.dartmouthatlas.org (accessed May 5, 2011).
10. Deming W.E.: *Out of the Crisis.* Boston: MIT Press, 1982.

11. Carey R.G., Lloyd R.C.: *Measuring Quality Improvement in Healthcare: A Guide to Statistical Process Control Applications.* Milwaukee, WI: ASQ Press, 2001.
12. Kolb D.A.: *Experiential Learning: Experience as the Source of Learning and Development.* Upper Saddle River, NJ: Prentice-Hall, 1984.
13. Nelson E.C., Batalden P.B., Lazar J.S. (eds.): *Practice-Based Learning and Improvement: A Clinical Improvment Action Guide,* 2nd ed. Oak Brook, IL: Joint Commission Resources, 2007.
14. Nelson E.C., et al.: Report cards or instrument panels: Who needs what? *Jt Comm J Qual Improv* 21:155–166, Apr. 1995.

CHAPTER 7

Measurement Part 2: Using Run Charts and Statistical Process Control Charts to Gain Insight into Systems

OBJECTIVES

After reading this chapter, you will be able to do the following:

1. Recognize the value of analyzing data over time by using run charts and statistical process control charts.
2. Describe the difference between common cause variation and special cause variation.
3. Interpret run charts and statistical process control charts.

Jonah Mills has been a family physician in rural Idaho for more than 12 years. He recently assumed responsibility as the medical director for three family medicine clinics. It has been a challenging transition. The clinics are located in different towns in the region, about 20–30 minutes from one another, and Jonah has been trying to unify their approach to patient care. Today Jonah is meeting with the multisite quality improvement team, which includes nurses, physician assistants, an office administrator, students, and other physicians, to review some recent data about the treatment for heart failure at all three facilities.

The three clinics initiated an electronic health record (EHR) system about one year ago. There was—as would be expected—a significant learning period to integrate the new technology into patient care. Initially, it was challenging just to find information and enter it into patient charts. One advantage of this particular EHR system is that the software provider was able to download patient data from the prior lab and pharmacy records. Although the EHR system has been in use for only about a year, the database contains patient data from the past several years.

The team reviewed the data on heart failure. While almost every patient has had an echocardiogram to assess left ventricular function, the team is concerned about the low rate of beta-blocker use for patients with heart failure (see Table 7-1 below). Research evidence shows that the use of beta-blockers is associated with a significant increase in left ventricular function and a decrease in mortality. Jonah is not sure what to make of the data and asks the team, "When you look at these numbers from our three sites, which site has the 'best' outcomes? Who's made the most gains over the past year? Who needs the most help?"

QI Measurement—Evaluating Systems over Time

Chapter 6 discusses the historical developments of measuring outcomes in clinical care and also provides tools for identifying measures for a clinical system. This chapter focuses on using methods to measure systems in health care in order to gain insight

TABLE 7-1.

Percentage of Patients with Heart Failure Who Were Receiving a Beta-Blocker

Month	Site 1	Site 2	Site 3
January 2009	31%	44%	33%
February 2009	38	45	30
March 2009	35	41	31
April 2009	40	45	29
May 2009	32	36	31
June 2009	35	39	32
July 2009	30	46	33
August 2009	36	48	35
September 2009	38	40	38
October 2009	35	46	44
November 2009	31	49	46
December 2009	35	46	45
January 2010	36	44	44
February 2010	35	43	48
March 2010	36	41	49
April 2010	37	41	50
May 2010	38	40	49
June 2010	42	39	48
July 2010	50	38	47
August 2010	37	41	49
September 2010	35	39	48
October 2010	31	38	48
November 2010	34	39	50
December 2010	33	37	47
2009 average	35%	44%	36%
2010 average	37%	40%	48%

into the functioning of the system. We will focus on a dynamic form of measurement intended to monitor systems for changes that occur and to predict what will happen in the future: the run chart and the control chart.

Measurement for improvement is different from other forms of measurement. Unlike most traditional statistics, measurement for improvement is not intended to identify differences between groups (static, one point in time) but is intended to monitor systems over time (dynamic, continuous measurement). Most traditional data analyses look backward and reflect what has been measured in the past, like looking out the side mirror in a car (*see* Figure 7-1 on page 100).[1] While these analyses provide a sufficient summary of where you have been, they provide only a slight view of what lies ahead (perhaps like looking around the edges of the side mirror). In contrast, analyzing data over time—with the use of run charts and control charts—offers a much different perspective; it is like looking out the front window of a car while driving (*see* Figure 7-2 on page 100). When you are looking out the front window, the mirror provides a panoramic view of the road behind; however, you also see a clear view out the front window, allowing you to anticipate the road ahead. Similarly, analyzing data over time can identify how a system is currently operating and even predict future functioning of the system. These tools provide a statistically powerful method to understand what is happening in a system.

For example, imagine that an intensive care unit (ICU) improvement team is evaluating the outcome of the initiation of a bundled intervention to reduce ventilator-associated pneumonia (VAP).[2,3] A *bundle* is a group of evidence-based interventions that are known to improve outcomes and should be implemented together for maximum effectiveness.[4] The team began implementing the VAP bundle in January 2010. In January 2011 the chief quality officer wants to know whether the bundle intervention has made a difference. The team uses two approaches: traditional statistics, using a before-and-after comparison of average number of infections and monthly data displayed on a run chart. In the table in Figure 7-3 on page 101, the traditional summary statistics demonstrate a decrease from an average of seven infections per month in 2009 to an average of two infections per month in 2010. It is encouraging that such a dramatic change is seen even without running a specific statistical test. However, when the team uses a dynamic display of data in a run chart, it is clear that the reduction in VAP started prior to the bundle implementation (note the trend that started in July and August 2009). It appears that since the intervention of the bundle, the rate of VAP has been steady. The improvement team notes that further analysis may be needed to determine whether the bundle was effective in maintaining the lower rate of infections. Perhaps the bundle helped the unit reach zero infections in April and November 2010? As discussed in Chapter 6, summary data in a static, tabular format are not effective for assessing the impact of interventions.

FIGURE 7-1. *Traditional Statistics Provide a Clear View of Past Performance**

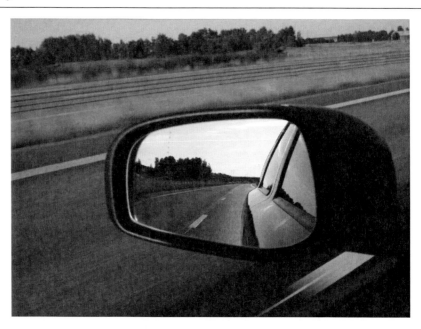

* As with a side mirror in a car, with traditional statistics, you mostly see the road behind, with a bit of the road ahead around the edges.

FIGURE 7-2. *Examining Data over Time: A View of Past Performance with an Expectation About Future Performance**

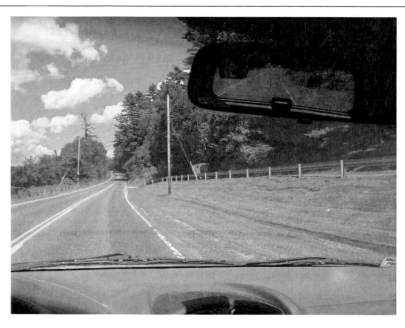

* As with a view out the front window of a car, with data examined over time (using run charts and control charts), you see the road ahead as well as a clear picture of what is behind you.

Run Charts and Statistical Process Control Charts: The Basics

A defining characteristic of quality improvement is to show that the strategy for change (which is often multifaceted) works to bring about a measurable difference in process or outcome. Two-point before–after studies provide weak demonstrations of change. Strong demonstrations of change overcome the limitation of before–after analysis by capitalizing on the concept of replication. *Replication*, or the process of evaluating successive results, shows that an intervention produces the pattern of change observed in the results. Run charts and statistical process control (SPC) charts (sometimes simply called *control charts*) use the principle of replication for analysis to demonstrate whether a change has occurred from preintervention (baseline phase) to postintervention (implementation phase). These charts are within the family of time-series analyses that plot multiple points, with each point representing the operationally defined unit of measurement (such as a daily, weekly, or monthly proportion or mean or time between events).[5]

Run charts and statistical process control (SPC) charts (sometimes simply called control charts) use the principle of replication for analysis to demonstrate whether a change has occurred from preintervention (baseline phase) to postintervention (implementation phase).

FIGURE 7-3. *Comparison of Yearly Summary Data and Monthly Data, Graphed over Time for Ventilator-Associated Pneumonia (VAP) in the Intensive Care Unit**

Evaluation of Ventilator-Associated Pneumonia in the ICU, 2009–2011		
Year	Total Number of VAP Cases	Average VAP Cases
2009	85	7
2010	24	2

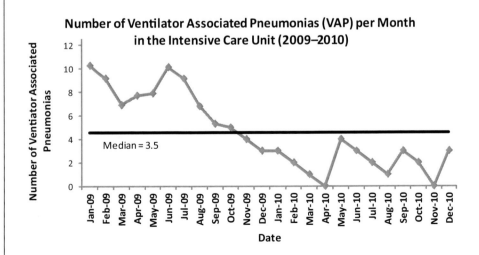

* The arrow indicates when the bundle intervention was initiated at the start of 2010. Notice that the decrease in VAP started in September 2009, before the bundle was initiated.

Analyzing Why a Significant System Change Occurs

When a run chart or an SPC chart has at least 14 data points, the probability of a special cause "signal" is less than 5% (equivalent to p value < 0.05). This is based on probability statistics of replication, which generate power from point-to-point variation in order to detect a signal. So, when a signal appears in a chart, it is the same power as a p value < 0.05 that occurs in traditional statistics. These methods can detect that a statistically significant change has occurred in a system, but a team must identify *why* it has occurred: a new process, a reaction to a change to the system, stress on the system from an external source (for example, many staff out sick). Evaluating a system with these tools identifies *what* has occurred in the system and gives the team the opportunity to gain insight into *why* the system responded as it did.

How Run Charts Work

A run chart displays data in a time-ordered sequence (*see* Figures 7-4a and 7-4b on page 103) and can easily be constructed with graph paper and a pencil. Time is plotted along the *x*-axis, and the appropriate scale for the data is used for the *y*-axis. The time on the *x*-axis may be days, months, or quarters, or it may consist of consecutive measurements (for example, blood sugar, blood pressure) taken over some time period, even if not done at regularly spaced intervals. The body of the run chart contains the values in consecutive order, connected by a line. As the data are plotted on the run chart, a measure of central tendency is also added. For a run chart, the measure of central tendency is the median, the point at which half of the data points are above the line and half of the data points are below the line. For example, in a run chart with 25 data points, as in Figure 7-4a, the median line would be drawn at a location where 12 data points are above the line and 12 data points are below it (the median is 121 in this example). Run charts can be used for any process and with any type of data: whole numbers, percentages, proportions.

How Control Charts Work

A statistical process control chart uses point-to-point variation in data to derive control limits. The most essential type of SPC is an XmR chart that uses the average as the measure of central tendency (*see* Figure 7-5 on page 104). The upper control limit (UCL) and lower control limit (LCL) represent boundaries that are about three standard deviations on each side of the average. These are calculated using a formula that includes the average of the data points (x), the average of the difference between each data point (R), and a constant (2.66). It is represented as follows:

$$UCL = x + 2.66*R$$
$$LCL = x - 2.66*R$$

Thus, as each new point is added to the chart, the average, UCL, and LCL are updated. This is the important dynamic characteristic mentioned earlier in the chapter. Because these calculations change with each point that is added, control charts are often constructed with the help of computer software.

FIGURE 7-4. *Anatomy of a Run Chart**

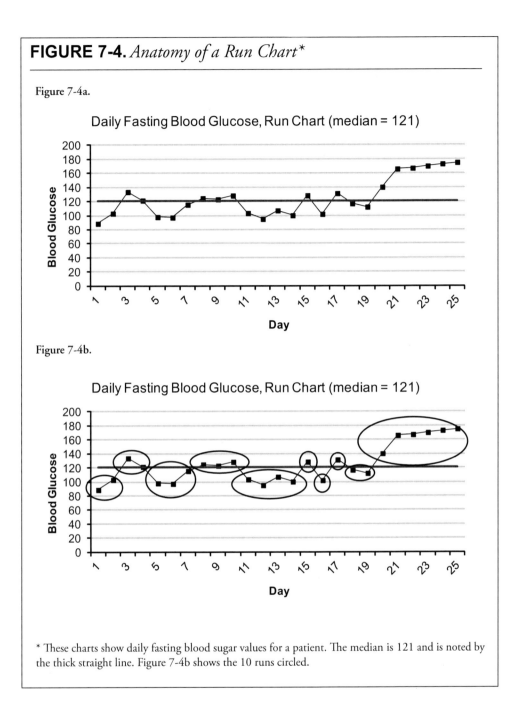

Figure 7-4a.

Figure 7-4b.

* These charts show daily fasting blood sugar values for a patient. The median is 121 and is noted by the thick straight line. Figure 7-4b shows the 10 runs circled.

The basic anatomy of a control chart is similar to that of a run chart. Time is represented on the *x*-axis, and the data values are on the *y*-axis. Individual data points are plotted in the body of the figure. The average and the control limits are derived from the data. The data in Figure 7-5 are the same as in the run chart in Figure 7-4a, but notice that the average in the control chart is 125, while the median in the run chart is 121. The added power of a control chart comes from the UCL and LCL, which are 162 and 88 in Figure 7-5. These control limits provide the parameters that begin to explain the variation in the data.

FIGURE 7-5. *Anatomy of a Control Chart**

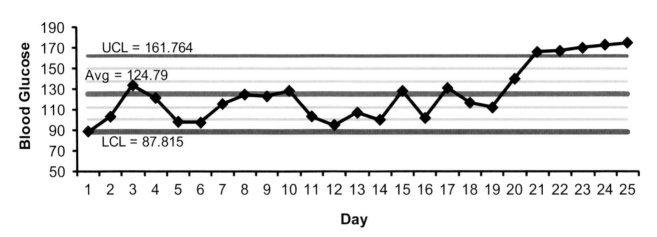

Daily Fasting Blood Glucose, XmR Chart, average = 124.8

* This chart shows daily fasting blood sugar values for a patient. The mean is 124.8 (middle line), the upper control limit (UCL) is 161.8, and the lower control limit (LCL) is 87.8.

Common Cause Variation and Special Cause Variation

Whether using run charts or control charts to represent data, determining the type of variation present in data is a vital step in taking the correct action. There are two types of variation to understand: common cause variation and special cause variation. Common cause variation is considered inherent in a process and due to regular, natural, or ordinary causes. It usually affects all the outcomes and steps of a process and results in a stable process that is predictable. Sometimes this is called *random*, or *unassignable*, *variation*. Special cause variation is due to effects that are usually outside the steps of the process. This variation often affects some, but not necessarily all, aspects of the process and results in an unstable, unpredictable process. Special cause variation is sometimes called *nonrandom*, or *assignable*, *variation*.

Common cause variation does not mean "good" variation. It only means that the process is stable and predictable. Similarly, special cause variation does not mean "bad" variation. A special cause may represent a very good result, which you might want to enhance. *Special cause* merely means that something has affected the process to make it unstable and unpredictable. For example, imagine that you are seeing a patient with high blood pressure who is measuring his pressure at home every day. Over the course of two weeks, his systolic blood pressure ranges from 158 to 173 mmHg. This two-week block of data would indicate entirely common cause variation. The blood pressure is stable and predictable, and the data contain only common cause variation; however, the results are entirely unacceptable because the goal of systolic blood pressure is less than 140 mmHg. You introduce an antihypertensive medication

---

DEFINED:
Common and Special Cause Variations

Common cause variation is considered inherent in a process and due to regular, natural, or ordinary causes. Special cause variation is due to effects that are usually outside the steps of the process.

Sidebar 7-1. *Demonstrating Common Cause Variation and Special Cause Variation*

One way to examine the difference between common cause variation and special cause variation is with a simple and often-used classroom exercise. In this example, a class of 22 students used 1.69-ounce packages of chocolates coated with green, red, blue, yellow, orange, and brown candy shells. One bag was given to each student so that he or she could use statistical process control to develop a way to predict the number of green candies in each bag. Students opened their bags one at a time, and they counted the number of green candies. Using a spreadsheet, the class created a run chart of the data (*see* Figure 7-6a below). When all 22 students had submitted their data, the data were plotted on an XmR control chart (*see* Figure 7-6b below). The control limits were the parameters within which the students could then predict the number of green candies in unopened packages. The students then opened five more bags of candies, and sure enough, the number of green candies in bags 23 through 26 fell within the predicted range of 4 to 18 (the LCL and UCL of 3.9 and 17.8, respectively). The interpretation of these charts (*see* Figures 7-6a and 7-6b below) indicated only common cause variation. There were no special cause signals. The system for green candies in a package was stable and predictable.

FIGURE 7-6.

Figure 7-6a. Run chart of the number of green candies in each bag.

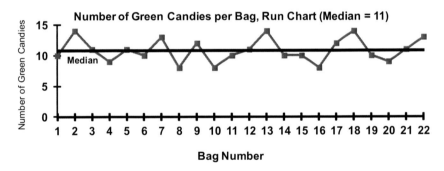

Figure 7-6b. XmR control chart of the number of green candies in each bag.

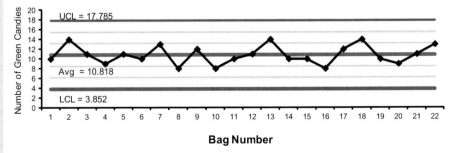

(continued)

Sidebar 7-1. *Demonstrating Common Cause Variation and Special Cause Variation* (continued)

Next, the class opened a 1.69-ounce package of holiday candies containing only green and red candies. How many green candies did that package contain? Twenty-five. The addition of the holiday package to the series served as an example of a special cause variation. It indicated a change in the underlying production process (that is, the underlying system). Figure 7-6c below shows the addition of bags 23–26 and the holiday bag, point 27. This point is above the UCL, indicating that there is special cause variation. In this case, the reason for the special cause signal was obvious: a different production of candies for the holidays. As you will see later, identifying special cause variation directs you to examine the process and system from which the data arise to identify the source of the special cause.

Figure 7-6c. XmR control chart of the number of green candies from a holiday package of candies. Notice that point 27 is above the upper control limit, indicating a special cause signal.

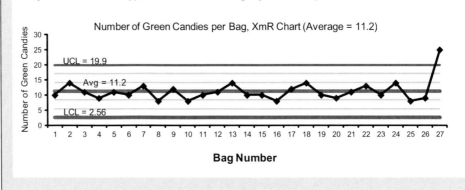

to this patient. Over the course of several days, his systolic blood pressure drops to between 125 and 140 mmHg. This would be considered a special cause variation as it is a significant disruption to the system, but it is a good special cause variation. The blood pressure system for this patient at this point in time is considered unstable and unpredictable, even though it has been moved closer to the clinical goal.

Implications of Differences in Causes of Variation

The key point is that knowledge of a process and a system helps you identify whether the outcomes are acceptable. In measurement for improvement—whether for high blood pressure in an individual patient or the percentage of patients with controlled high blood pressure in a microsystem—the measures become part of the feedback process and may influence the changes in the system.

Determining whether variation is due to special or common causes has profound implications for whether and how you should take action on a system. Recall in Chapter 6 how understanding the variation in Mary and Bill's target shooting (*see* Figure 6-4 in Chapter 6) guided how each would change his or her approach in order to hit the bull's eye consistently. Understanding the type of variation in your data (and thus in your system) directs you to take appropriate action on the system (*see* Table 7-2 below). If action is needed in a system and you indeed take action, this is the appropriate step to take. Similarly, if action is *not* needed and action is *not* taken, this is also appropriate. Systemic losses in efficacy and efficiency occur when action is needed but not taken. This leads to loss of efficacy and efficiency from passivity. Similarly, if action is *not* needed but is taken—for example, if many changes are made to a process without understanding the underlying variation—the system experiences loss of efficacy and efficiency from tampering. Understanding the variation in the data leads to better improvement and substantial insight into the process, which leads to more effective change.

Interpreting Run Charts and Control Charts

Using a run chart is the simplest way to analyze data over time. In many ways, the run chart is the forerunner of the control chart. Either chart can assist in determining the type of variation present in a system, but in some ways, a run chart is similar to a plain x-ray, while a control chart is similar to a CT scan. An x-ray is often simpler to obtain and interpret but gives less information than a CT scan. Sometimes an x-ray is all that is needed to make a diagnosis; however, other times, the additional time, detail, and expense of the CT scan is required for the appropriate diagnosis and treatment of a patient. Similarly, a run chart may be appropriate for a simple and straightforward analysis of a system, but sometimes a control chart is needed for more detailed and in-depth analysis.

Interpreting each run chart and control chart aids in understanding data. There are rules of detection to identify special cause variation in these charts. If none of the rules are fulfilled, then the chart indicates only common cause variation. These rules are based on probability that certain patterns would not occur by chance alone. Let us look at each of the basic rules of detection and illustrate with a few examples.

TABLE 7-2.
Deciding Whether to Take Action*

		What do you do?	
		Action taken	Action **not** taken
What signal(s) come from the control chart?	Action needed	✓	**Loss from passivity**
	Action **not** needed	**Loss from tampering**	✓

* Examining data over time with a run chart or control chart will help you determine whether action is needed. Taking action on a system that is stable is tampering and will likely lead to loss of efficiency and effectiveness. Similarly, *not* taking action on a system that is out of control is passive and leads to a loss of efficiency and effectiveness.

Rules of Detection in Run Charts

A run chart should have at least 14 points in order to have sufficient power to draw conclusions. The example in Figure 7-4a has 25 points of daily fasting blood sugar data for a patient with diabetes, so there is adequate power to proceed with interpretation. Three rules of detection are applied to each run chart to determine whether the chart shows any of the following special cause signals:

1. Too few or too many runs, which is an assessment of the overall variability in the data

2. A shift in the process with seven or more consecutive points on one side of the median

3. A trend of seven or more points continually increasing or decreasing

The presence of any one of these signals indicates a change in the data (and a change in the process that the data represent) that is statistically significant.

Special cause signal 1—Indication of overall variability. Too few or too many runs are determined by counting the number of runs on a chart. A *run* is a group of successive points (or even one point) on one side of the median. If a point falls on the median, it is not counted as part of a run because it does not add further information about variability in the data. The number of runs is an estimate of the overall variability in the data, determined from probability statistics, and is found in a statistical table that provides the low and high expected number of runs, based on the total number of points in a chart (*see* Table 7-3 on page 110).[6] A chart with 25 points should have between 9 and 17 runs. If there were fewer than 9, it would be a special cause signal of too little variability. If there were more than 17, it would be a special cause signal of too much variability. The example in Figure 7-4b has each run circled. There are 10 runs total, so the amount of overall variability is appropriate; there is no special cause from signal 1.

Special cause signal 2—Indication of a shift in the process. The second test is for a shift in the process. A shift occurs when there are 7 or more consecutive points on one side of the median. There is no shift in Figure 7-4a.

Special cause signal 3—Indication of a trend. The third test is for a trend, which is indicated by at least 7 consecutive points increasing or decreasing. One increasing trend is present in Figure 7-4a, from day 19 through day 25, indicating a signal of special cause variation.

Determining the reason variation has occurred. Although a run chart can identify variation, it does not tell you *why* the variation has occurred. For example, we identified a trend in Figure 7-4a, indicating a special cause signal that something has perturbed this patient's self-care system. To determine why this has occurred, we need to turn to the process of care for this patient. Upon further investigation, we find that this patient was on vacation and was not able to follow his diabetic diet while traveling. He ate more sweets and carbohydrates than usual during that time period. The run chart gives us the power to identify that the change in dietary intake was significant enough to cause a real, statistical change in the patient's fasting blood sugar. This was not just a slight bump from being on vacation but rather indicates a significant change to his self-care system.

Rules of Detection in Control Charts

Like a run chart, a control chart should have at least 14 points in order to have sufficient power to draw conclusions; however; the UCL and LCL provide additional ways to test for special causes of variation. In control charts, runs are not counted because the width of the control limits (that is, the distance between the LCL and the UCL) estimates the overall variability. Very wide control limits indicate more variability than narrow control limits. Special cause variation is identified when one of the following signals occurs:

1. A single point falling outside a control limit
2. A shift in the process, with seven or more consecutive points on one side of the median
3. A trend of seven or more points continually increasing or decreasing

After the data are plotted on a control chart (using the formulas from page 102 or computer software), the rules for detecting special cause variation are applied. The control chart in Figure 7-5 is an XmR chart that contains the same trend from day 19 through 25 that is observed in Figure 7-4a. There are no shifts in the control chart; however, with the addition of the control limits, we can identify a special cause on the third point of the trend on Day 21. This is the first point outside the control limits. Had we observed these points as they occurred each morning, we could have identified a significant change in the patient's fasting blood sugar (on Day 21) several days earlier with the control chart than with the run chart; we would have found it on Day 25, the seventh point in the trend.

Acting on Interpretations from the Charts

Run charts and control charts are tools to help us focus on taking the correct action. The action for the diabetic patient in our example is guided by the insight garnered from the charts. The patient and his health care team are now aware that vacations are a time when he needs more support for his diabetes care. Perhaps a refresher session with a diabetes dietary counselor about healthy eating while traveling would be helpful. Maybe he requires a short-term increase in his medications. The special cause signal directs specific actions to bring the system into control in order to meet the goal.

But what if there were no special cause signals? The interpretation would then be that the chart shows only common cause variation. The action to address common cause variation is quite different. Instead of addressing specific issues such as dietary intake while on vacation, the provider and patient would examine the overall system performance, determine whether the patient is meeting his goal, and, if he is not

TABLE 7-3.

Determining the Expected Number of Runs

Number of Data Points Not on the Median	Lowest Run Count	Highest Run Count
12	3	10
13	4	10
14	4	11
15	4	12
16	5	12
17	5	13
18	6	13
19	6	14
20	6	15
21	7	15
22	7	16
23	8	16
24	8	17
25	9	17
26	9	18
27	9	19
28	10	19
29	10	20
30	11	20

at goal, then address the underlying processes of diabetes care for the patient. If he were at goal, then no changes would be the appropriate course of action. If he were not at the goal, the processes of diabetes care need to be addressed—for example, carbohydrate intake, daily exercise regimen, and medication dosages.

Using Control Charts to Predict Future Performance

Another advantage of the control chart is that the control limits can help predict future performance (*see* Figure 7-2). Over the past 25 days, the UCLs and LCLs for our scenario patient's fasting blood sugar have been between 87 and 162. Using the predictive characteristics of a control chart, we anticipate this person to have a fasting blood sugar between 87 and 162. When each value is added to the chart, the control limits adjust; this is the dynamic property of a control chart. The chart is continually updated to account for the new information that arrives with each new data point. Although this patient can anticipate fairly good blood sugar control (between 87 and 162 fasting blood sugar), as soon as the 164 blood sugar occurs on Day 21, the chart would prompt the patient to realize that this is unusual, enabling him to determine the cause and take action.

Control Limits for Groups of Data

Another feature of the control chart is that control limits can be used for groups of data in a chart. In other words, one chart may have data with two sets of control limits. For example, to evaluate the effectiveness of an intervention, control limits for the process before the intervention can be held constant, and new control limits can be recalculated, reflecting the time after the intervention is implemented. This is called *splitting* the control limits. Another example of this is when there is a long run of data that is outside the control limit. The data prior to this special cause variation can be held constant and new control limits calculated. (*See* the continuation of the vignette that follows for an example where this would be appropriate.) Splitting and recalculating control limits helps to determine when special cause variation becomes stable at a new level (that is, it now becomes new common cause variation), another example of the dynamic nature of control charts.

XmR Control Charts

There are many different types of control charts to use. The most common is the XmR chart, which is robust enough to be used with any type of data. In addition to XmR charts, other specific control charts can be used, depending on the underlying distribution of the data (for example, normal, binomial, geometric). The calculations used in the XmR chart make it strong enough to be used with any data that have any underlying distribution. While other types of charts might technically be more appropriate for percentage or proportion data, an XmR chart is valid for plotting almost any data. For more detailed information about control charts in health care settings, see the books by Carey[6] and Wheeler[7] or the article by Amin[8] listed at the end of this chapter.

Now let's return to our example of the improvement team concerned about the low rate of beta-blocker use for patients with heart failure to see how the concepts we have discussed come together.

The team comments that it is difficult to determine which site is performing best using the data. In Table 7-1, it appears that Site 2 was the best performer in 2009. It regressed a bit in 2010. Sites 1 and 3 were about equal in 2009, but Site 3 made a spectacular 12% increase over the year. The team suggests examining the data in a more comprehensive way; it considers using all the data for the past 24 months to create run and control charts.

Jonah Mills has the data in two formats. First, the team examines the data using run charts (see Figures 7-7a through 7-7c on page 112). Although Table 7-1 shows that Site 3 had the best performance, the team agrees that from the run charts, it is clear that much of that site's improvement occurred more than 14 months ago! The team applies the rules for detecting

FIGURE 7-7. *Run Charts of the Percentage of Beta-Blocker Use by Patients with Heart Failure by Site, 2009–2010*

Figure 7-7a. Site 1

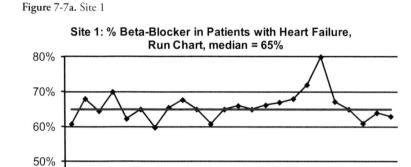

Figure 7-7b. Site 2

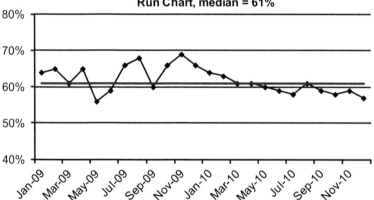

Figure 7-7c. Site 3

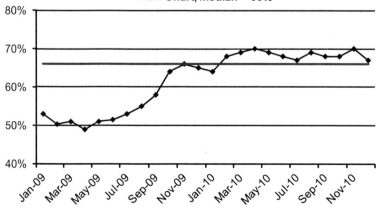

special cause variation and finds too few runs in the chart for Site 3 (only two), which indicates a special cause occurring at Site 3. Similarly, Site 2, which initially had the best performance and then declined, shows a trend that occurred from November to July. This is a special cause signal, and the process that produced that result should be investigated. Finally, Site 1 remained just about the same over the 24 months. There was a peak in July 2010, but on the run chart, this is common cause variation. The team summarizes its analysis in a table (see Table 7-4 below).

Jonah is impressed with the team's analytical ability, and he turns now to the XmR control charts, which contain the same data used before (see Figures 7-8a to 7-8c on page 114). Examining the data using the control charts, the team notices that Site 1 had a special cause signal in July 2010. Site 2 has the same trend seen in the run chart and also shows a shift (March–September 2010). Site 3 is most striking, and nursing student Kaitlyn Smith states, "This is interesting [pointing at Figure 7-8c]: Site 3 did so much better after it implemented an intervention in October of 2009 to improve beta-blocker use. But it seems that the effect was limited, and the system has been stable since then. It's hard to see with the control limits as they are drawn. Can we adjust the chart to make this change more apparent?"

Jonah appreciates Kaitlyn's insight and shows the team a chart with the control limits split and recalculated (see Figure 7-8d). "Essentially, the system has remained stable for the past 14 months. It now has an average of about 67.5% of patients receiving beta-blockers but can expect to operate anywhere from 63.4% to 71.5% over the next few months unless something is done to change the system. Kaitlyn comments, "It's unfortunate that Site 3 made such good progress and then leveled off and has not continued to improve the system since October 2009."

TABLE 7-4.
Summary Interpretation of the Run Charts from Sites 1–3
(Figures 7-7a–7-7c)*

Site	Number of runs	Shift?	Trend?	Interpretation	Action
1	9	No	No	Common cause variation	Will need to examine the fundamental process of beta-blocker prescribing.
2	6	No	Yes	Two special cause signals	Investigate the trend to determine why the decrease in performance occurred at that time.
3	2	Yes	Yes	Three special cause signals	Investigate all three signals to determine why the site has leveled off in performance.

* From Table 7-3, the expected number of runs is between 8 and 17.

FIGURE 7-8. *XmR Control Charts of the Percentage of Beta-Blocker Use by Patients with Heart Failure by Site, 2009–2010*

Figure 7-8a. Site 1

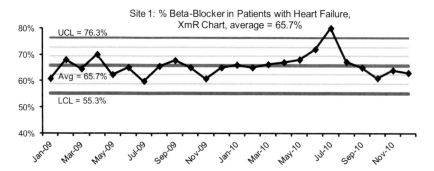

Figure 7-8b. Site 2

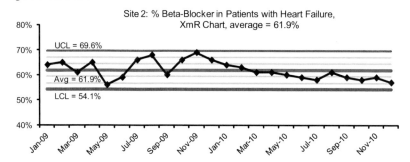

Figure 7-8c. Site 3

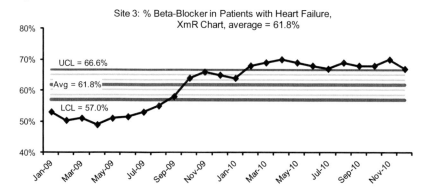

Figure 7-8d. Site 3 (split and recalculated)

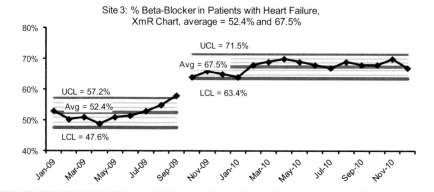

TABLE 7-5.

Summary Interpretation of the XmR Control Charts from Sites 1–3 (Figures 7-8a–7-8d)

Site	LCL	UCL	Points Outside the Control Limits?	Shift?	Trend?	Interpretation	Action
						Original Control Limits	
1	55.3	76.3	One	No	No	One special cause signal	Investigate the point above the UCL from July 2010. What went right this month?
2	54.1	69.6	No	Yes	Yes	Two special cause signals	Investigate the decreasing trend to determine why the performance changed and remained at a lower level.
3	57.0	66.6	Many	Yes	Yes	Three special cause signals	Investigate all three signals as to why the site has leveled off in performance.
						Recalculated Control Limits	
3	47.6	57.2	One	No	No	One special cause signal	None because it was in the distant past.
	63.4	71.5	No	No	No	Common cause variation in past 14 months	Examine the fundamental process of beta-blocker prescribing. How can we move to even better performance? Why are we "stuck" at 67.5%?

Jonah pauses and considers the other XmR charts (see Figures 7-8a and 7-8b). "In many ways," he says, "this is equally cause for concern: Site 2 had some episodes of increasing its numbers, but the past 12 months have seen a decrease, with 10 consecutive months under the center line. It is concerning that the system has taken a downward turn, and this should be addressed soon. Site 1 is interesting: In July 2010, it reached 80% of patients. This is above the UCL of 76.3%, so it is a special cause. I wonder what happened that month to get such good results. And why the decline since then?" The team summarizes the analysis in a table (see Table 7-5 above).

He continues, "We've all been trying hard to improve and have shown some successes. These charts help us identify where the changes have made a real difference and how we may amplify their successes and perhaps reverse trends where the outcomes are not as strong as we want." The team agrees and determines that the next step is to meet with the individual clinic directors to discuss the control chart results.

Summary

A defining characteristic of quality improvement is to demonstrate that the strategy for change works to bring about a measurable difference in process or outcome. Measurement for improvement monitors systems and processes over time (dynamic, continuous measurement); whereas traditional statistics are usually used to identify differences between groups (static, cross-sectional). The two main measurement tools are run charts and statistical process control charts. Run charts and control charts use the principle of replication to demonstrate whether a change has occurred from preintervention (baseline phase) to postintervention (implementation phase).

Applying the rules for interpretation can help determine whether the variation in a process is due to common or special causes. These rules include identification of runs, trends, and out-of-control points. The interpretation of this variability directs *action* on the processes of a system. Measurement for improvement and the interpretation of the variability in processes or outcomes is a key to the success of quality improvement efforts in health care.

Study Questions

You are a member of your unit's cardiothoracic surgery quality improvement team. Surgery has always been fascinating to you, and heart and lung surgery is the most interesting of all. You enjoy the clinical work, and this hospital is a new member of a regional consortium that is focused on improving all aspects of their coronary artery bypass graft (CABG) surgeries. What an opportunity to combine your love of surgery as a discipline and learn to improve care for surgical patients!

Throughout the first week, you notice that the team waits for a serum potassium level before the patient can come off the heart/lung bypass machine. This is important because patients who are on the bypass machine for a longer period have more complications. In the first six cases this week, it has taken between 12 and 40 minutes for the "stat" potassium level to be reported by the lab. Everyone in the operating room (OR) "knows that the lab is slow," but you wonder what is really happening with this process.

One morning later this week, the first case of the day for your team is canceled. Instead of catching up on some reading, you decide to follow a stat potassium sample from the other OR to the lab and back. You make some notes and create a deployment-type flowchart of the sample's journey (see Figure 7-9 on page 117).

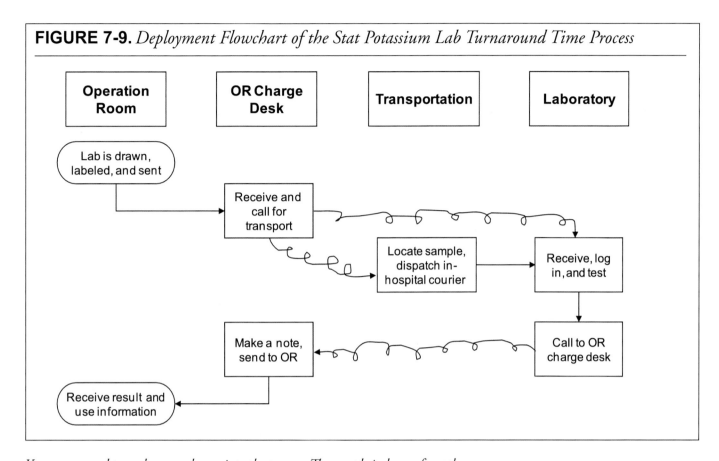

FIGURE 7-9. *Deployment Flowchart of the Stat Potassium Lab Turnaround Time Process*

You are amazed to see how much goes into the process. The sample is drawn from the patient in the OR and taken to the OR charge desk, where the surgical clerk, who seems to do everything for everyone at the same time (and does a good job of it), calls for a transport. Once in the chemistry lab, the sample is logged, run, and completed within about seven minutes. The lab has very clear records of this. The result is then telephoned back to the surgical clerk, who may or may not be able to answer the phone and relay the lab result to the OR right away. You draw curlicue-style lines to show where there are significant delays and variability in the process. Wow! What a complicated process for such a seemingly simple lab test!

You decide to collect data to evaluate this process, so you go back through the last 30 CABG cases and create a control chart of the number of minutes for the stat potassium to be reported to the OR. Your initial XmR chart looks like the one shown in Figure 7-10 on page 118.

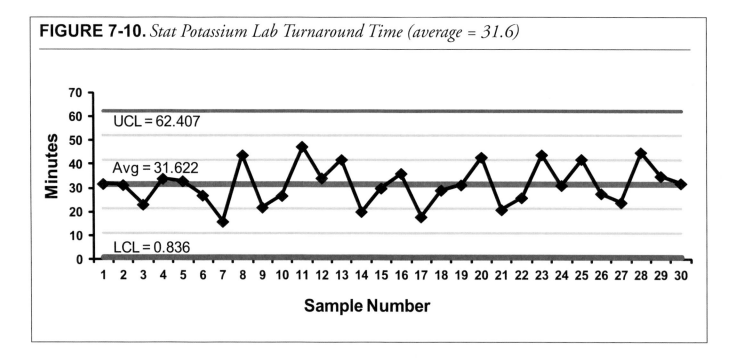

FIGURE 7-10. *Stat Potassium Lab Turnaround Time (average = 31.6)*

1. How can you use the information in the XmR chart shown in Figure 7-10 to describe the current system?
   a. Are there any signals that there may be special cause variation in the process?
   b. What does it mean to have common cause variation in this process?
   c. If no changes are made to the system, how long do you anticipate it would take for the next stat potassium sample to be reported?

After you review the process diagram and the chart with the team, everyone is impressed with your knowledge and assessment of the system. One of the nurse anesthetists recommends that the lab call directly to the OR instead of relaying the message through the surgical clerk. The lab agrees to try this change for a week, and stat potassium turnaround times from the eight cases that week are added to the XmR chart (see Figure 7-11 on page 119).

2. What has happened to the performance of the system?
   a. Are there any signals that there may be special cause variation in the process?
   b. Is the system functioning at its goal of a stat potassium turnaround time of less than 15 minutes? How can you tell?
   c. What happened to the UCL and LCL? Why?
   d. What else does this chart tell you?

FIGURE 7-11. *Stat Potassium Lab Turnaround Time with Additional Eight Cases (average = 28.8)*

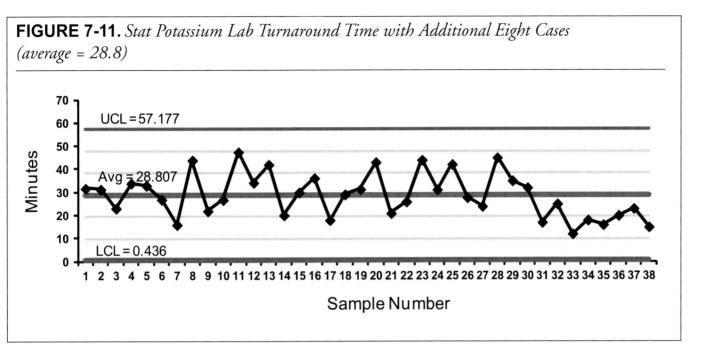

References

1. Wheeler D.J.: *Understanding Variation: The Key to Managing Chaos.* Knoxville, TN: SPC Press, 1993.
2. Rello J., et al.: A European care bundle for prevention of ventilator-associated pneumonia. *Intensive Care Med* 36:773–780, May, 2010.
3. Institute for Healthcare Improvement: *How-to Guide: Prevent Ventilator-Associated Pneumonia.* http://www.ihi.org/knowledge/Pages/Tools/HowtoGuidePreventVAP.aspx (accessed Sep. 30, 2011).
4. Institute for Healthcare Improvement: *What Is a Bundle?* http://www.ihi.org/knowledge/Pages/ImprovementStories/WhatIsaBundle.aspx (accessed Sep. 30, 2011).
5. Ogrinc G., et al.: The SQUIRE (Standards for QUality Improvement Reporting Excellence) guidelines for quality improvement reporting: Explanation and elaboration. *Qual Saf Health Care* 17(suppl. 1):i13–i32, Oct. 2008.
6. Carey R.G.: *Improving Health Care with Control Charts: Basic and Advanced SPC Methods and Case Studies.* Milwaukee: ASQ Quality Press, 2003.
7. Wheeler D.J.: *Making Sense of Data.* Knoxville, TN: SPC Press, 2003.
8. Amin S.G.: Control charts 101: A guide to health care applications. *Qual Manag Health Care* 9:1–27, Spring 2001.

CHAPTER 8

Understanding and Making Changes in a System

OBJECTIVES

After reading this chapter, you will be able to do the following:

1. Recognize that systems change occurs in a complex—not linear—fashion.
2. Identify the basic elements of a complex adaptive system.
3. Appropriately use Everett Rogers's description of adoption of innovation to target an intervention.
4. Identify barriers to change and how to address those barriers.
5. Describe the role and utility of the Plan–Do–Study–Act (PDSA) cycle methodology for testing small changes and for building knowledge about a system.

Bri'elle Wilson, a fourth-year medical student, is finishing her internal medicine outpatient rotation with physician Robert Jerome. She is ready to complete the rotation and move on to her residency interviews. She is looking forward to interviews for a general surgery residency and has been frustrated at what she perceives as the slow pace of outpatient general internal medicine.

She grabs the chart from the door of her next patient and scans the information. George Bernard is here for a hypertension follow-up. It has been challenging to get his blood pressure into the normal range over the past six months. He was initially 182/98. Robert, the physician, has added various antihypertensive medications from different classes, advised the patient on lifestyle changes, and increased several of the medications to maximum doses. Despite all this, Bri'elle notes that Mr. Bernard's blood pressure today is 156/86, still above the goal of < 140/< 90. She shakes her head in frustration, takes a deep breath to compose herself, knocks on the door, and enters the room.

Mr. Bernard is a 57-year-old welder who has been seeing Robert Jerome for about two years. Bri'elle introduces herself as a medical student, sits down, and says, "Thank you so much for coming today. I know you have been here about every six weeks or so, and it is sometimes difficult to come to the doctor that often. It looks like your blood pressure is still elevated today. What's your blood pressure been at home?"

Mr. Bernard shifts his weight in the chair, and says, "I'm not sure, doc. We've been adding medications and increasing medications, and I'm just not sure they're working. Is there something else we can do?" Bri'elle identifies an opportunity to educate the patient. She launches into a soliloquy about lifestyle changes (he is built for hypertension, being slightly obese with a round figure), weight loss, and alcohol and sodium intake effects on elevated blood pressure. She offers several bits of advice on how to decrease caloric intake by reducing portion size, stresses the importance of minimal to moderate alcohol consumption, and also identifies examples of high-salt foods. Mr. Bernard listens attentively and nods frequently. Bri'elle asks if he has any questions or any other concerns today. He replies that he does not, and she exits the room.

In the hallway, she catches up with Robert. The clinic nurse, Nancy Perez, also has the opportunity to join them in their discussion. Bri'elle relates her encounter with Mr. Bernard, and Robert nods knowingly. Nancy says, "He's been here twice in the past three months for blood pressure checks, and each time I have told him about losing weight and about decreasing his alcohol and salt intake. I'm not sure he understands. I've given him the handouts we made about healthy eating."

Robert looks frustrated. His expression reflects the feelings of both Bri'elle and Nancy. After a short pause, he says to Bri'elle, "Did you ask him whether he is taking all his medications as prescribed?" Bri'elle replies sheepishly, "I never got around to it; I was so intent on making sure I gave him the counseling that I thought he needed." "Let's go back in," Robert says, "and see him together. I wonder whether he's been taking all the meds and what factors might be contributing to his lifestyle choices."

The Complexity of Systems Changes

It may seem odd to start a chapter on systems change by describing an individual patient encounter. For most of this book, we have focused the aims, the process modeling, and the measurement on *systems of care* for populations of patients. So why do we now switch to a story of an individual patient to start the discussion of change? Recall the description of the levels of the health care system in Chapter 5, with the target diagram (*see* Figure 5-2 on page 63). It shows that at the center of every system in health care is the patient, in relation to his or her own self-care system. The frustration in this chapter's opening vignette is evident—the frustration of the medical student, the nurse, the physician, and the patient. We sometimes assume that the patient exists in isolation and that the changes in lifestyle and medication regimen we recommend will occur automatically when a patient exits the office. We "pull the lever" of adding a medication and expect an equal and simple reaction on the other end of the "machine"—in the life of the patient and in his or her physiology. In this case, the clinical team expected a lowering of Mr. Bernard's blood pressure. When we do not get the response we expect (for example, the blood pressure is still elevated, the patient's weight has increased a few pounds), we may be tempted to place the blame on the patient by saying that the patient is noncompliant with our recommendations.

The frustration and blame that we feel overlook the reality that the patient exists in a self-care system—at home, at work, at leisure. Many factors influence his or her self-care system: medication side effects and cost, family routines, the influence of friends and coworkers, knowledge about the disease process, and information from media and the Internet. All these factors affect the patient's decisions regarding what to eat, where to eat, what and where and how much to drink, and whether to take medications as prescribed. In contrast, clinicians often incorrectly assume that a simple "clinician recommendation/patient effect" relationship occurs predictably. This "one cause/one effect" relationship is a linear cause-and-effect sequence:

Patient with hypertension + Medication
= Patient with lower blood pressure from medication
or
Patient with hypertension + Education
= Patient with lower blood pressure from increased knowledge

While sometimes the relationship plays out in this aligned, sequential linear model, systems—even patient self-care systems—are usually not that simple; making changes to a system is complex.

Completing the Model for Improvement

This chapter completes the explanation of the Model for Improvement (*see* Figure 8-1 on page 124).[1] Sometimes improvement work starts when changes are made to a system without the foundational work of a clear aim, understanding of the processes, and identification of measures. Chapters 4 and 5 cover identifying an aim for improvement and modeling the process ("What are we trying to accomplish?"), and Chapters 6 and 7 explore measurement for improvement ("How will we know that a change is an improvement?"). We now turn our attention to making changes to improve care for patients.

The two-part final stage of the Model for Improvement. The final stage of the Model for Improvement has two parts: (1) "What changes can we make that will result in improvement?" and (2) the Plan–Do–Study–Act (PDSA) cycle. This two-step final stage allows an improvement team to first generate a list of possible changes that might be helpful (that is, brainstorm) and then to make small tests of these changes, using the PDSA methodology. Remaining faithful to the rigors of the Model for Improvement will confirm the aphorism that "all improvement requires change, but not all change leads to improvement."[2]

FIGURE 8-1. *The Model for Improvement*

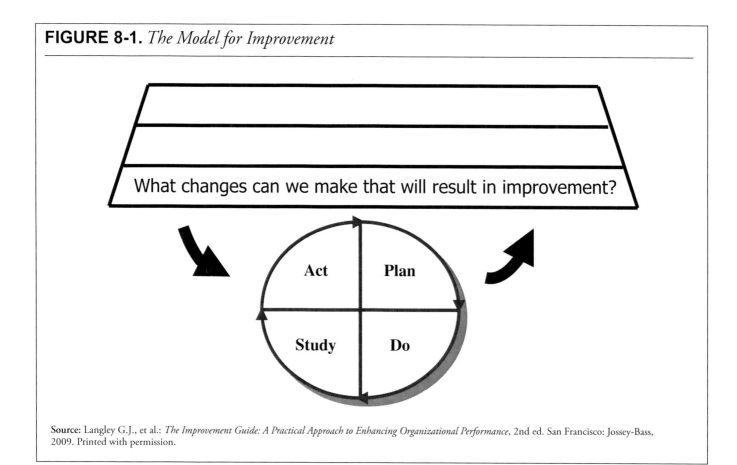

What changes can we make that will result in improvement?

Act | Plan
Study | Do

Source: Langley G.J., et al.: *The Improvement Guide: A Practical Approach to Enhancing Organizational Performance*, 2nd ed. San Francisco: Jossey-Bass, 2009. Printed with permission.

The evidence-based improvement equation applied to changes in a system. In Chapter 1 we introduced the evidence-based improvement equation (*see* Figure 8-2 on page 125).[3] This equation describes how the evidence that is derived from research is combined with the knowledge of systems and processes to achieve improved patient outcomes. In Chapter 1, we described the main components of this equation, but note here that the + and the → play a key role when considering changes in a system. The + is an indication of how the best evidence and the local setting are brought together. This is not a haphazard connection but requires a plan of change and a plan for linking the best evidence to the local practice. The → refers to executing the plan in the local setting. Executing the plan involves knowing the resources that are available to make it happen. The change must connect to the ways things work in this setting. Systems behave akin to biologic entities and rarely react in a linear fashion. In fact, systems react in an adaptive manner, so let us explore the properties of complex adaptive systems.

Complex Adaptive Systems

A *complex adaptive system (CAS)* is defined as "a collection of individual agents who have the freedom to act in ways that are not always predictable and whose actions are interconnected such that one agent's actions change the context for the other agents."[4(pp.312–313)] The study of CASs has been ongoing for more than 40 years, in fields

DEFINED: CAS

A complex adaptive system (CAS) is "a collection of individual agents who have the freedom to act in ways that are not always predictable and whose actions are interconnected such that one agent's actions change the context for the other agents."

FIGURE 8-2. *Evidence-Based Improvement Equation with Added Notations**

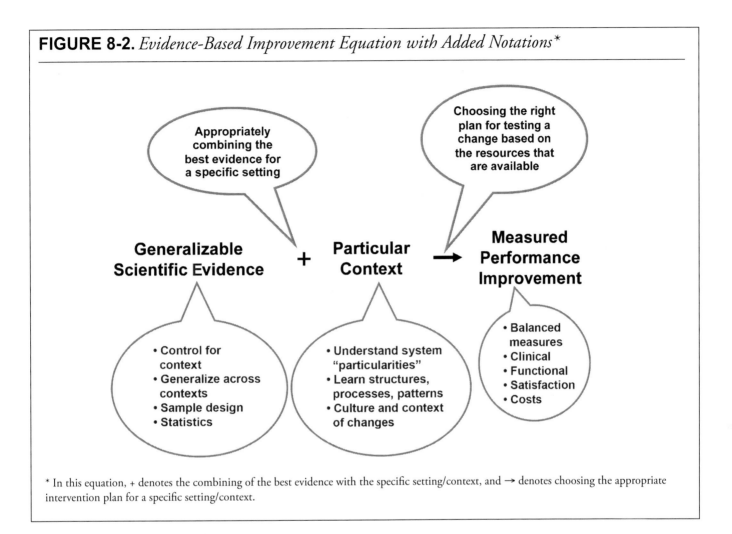

* In this equation, + denotes the combining of the best evidence with the specific setting/context, and → denotes choosing the appropriate intervention plan for a specific setting/context.

as diverse as immunology, biology (an ant colony is an example of a biological CAS), economics (the stock market is an example of an economic CAS), and sociology. Similarly, health care systems (at all levels) follow the principles of CASs. The "agents" in a CAS may be human or nonhuman, for the technology that is prevalent in health care also influences the system. Each agent's actions influence the *context* of the system, so understanding the context, culture, and processes of care are vital to understanding the nature of the CAS.

CAS Properties

There are eight principal properties of CASs that enable us to identify the components and interactions within the system. We will examine each of these and apply some of them to the self-care example from the opening vignette[4]:

1. **Adaptable elements:** In simple systems, machines and components must be changed by external forces; in CASs, the individual elements (whether antibiotic-resistant organisms or groups of people) can change on their own. The elements within a CAS have the internal capacity to change themselves.

2. **Simple rules:** The underlying norms that occur in a system may or may not be written down, but these norms act as rules that guide individual actions.

Although usually not lengthy, these rules provide guidance about how to act (and react) in relation to the other agents in the system.

3. **Nonlinear:** Because of interactions with the system, small changes may have very large effects, and large changes may have very small effects. For example, a hospital may initiate a new program with comprehensive training sessions for all its employees. Although this may be a massive effort, very little change might occur. In contrast, what initially seems like a small incident may have a large impact on how people perform their daily work.

4. **Novel:** Continual creativity is inherently part of the system. In a mechanical system such as an assembly line, actions are repetitive and predictable. In a CAS, the agents often try new ways to perform tasks.

5. **Unpredictable in detail:** Predicting the future is always challenging. The laws and rules that govern the movement of weather are helpful, but the interaction of those elements is complex, so accurate long-term forecasting is difficult. A complex system, such as weather, must be observed and monitored continually. This is the advantage of monitoring data over time, as discussed in Chapter 7. Run charts and statistical process control charts provide continual monitoring and display a degree of predictability in the systems.

6. **Inherently ordered:** Self-organization is a key idea in complexity science. For instance, there are no distinct rules that tell birds how and where to fly within a flock, yet birds are able to maintain a safe distance from one another and travel safely together.

7. **Contextual and embedded:** As we saw in the target diagram in Chapter 5, systems exist within systems and relate to other systems. In Chapter 5 we also discussed the importance of context and culture in a system for identifying the underlying elements that influence the functioning of the system. Although it is possible to identify the individual parts of a CAS, the reductionist approach is not as helpful as considering the fundamental wholeness of the system.

8. **Co-evolving:** The seven elements just described all contribute to a CAS moving forward through constant tension and then achieving a new balance. As a system is perturbed by change, the system achieves a new steady state. This holds true for single-celled organisms and also for large health care organizations. The tension, uncertainty, and anxiety that come with change are considered healthy elements in complex systems to achieve greater performance.

Applying the CAS Lens

Let's see how applying the CAS lens helps Robert and Bri'elle partner more effectively with Mr. Bernard.

Robert and Bri'elle enter Mr. Bernard's exam room, with a plan to focus on his alcohol intake as a modifiable factor to decrease his blood pressure. After some prompting, Mr. Bernard states, "Most of my alcohol intake is on weekends. I might have one to two beers at night during the week with my wife at dinner, but she doesn't enjoy drinking much. It's usually just the two of us for dinner. I often go out with friends from work on Friday night and have about six drinks or so. Also, Sunday afternoon is football time with my brothers, so probably another six drinks there."

From this brief reply, we learn a great deal about Mr. Bernard's alcohol intake—a focused element of the patient's self-care that directly affects his blood pressure. The *agents* in his self-care system include the patient himself, his spouse, his coworkers, and his brothers. Each of these individuals (and groups of individuals) is an independent *adaptable element*. There are some obvious *simple rules* that provide an *inherent order* that governs his interactions, such as "Football watching and alcohol are partners" and "Have only one or two drinks at home with my wife." His pattern and processes of alcohol consumption are *embedded* in the *context* of his life. Exactly how much Mr. Bernard drinks and when is probably *unpredictable in detail*. He may drink more if a certain coworker is present, or he may drink considerably less if his spouse accompanies him to watch the game on Sunday.

As the diagnosis of hypertension (and the effect of alcohol and antihypertensive medications) is superimposed upon Mr. Bernard's self-care system, it is easier to understand why he has not made lifestyle changes. What initially seemed like a straightforward "Decrease your alcohol consumption" lever is now viewed with the CAS lens. His complex adaptive personal care system might be affected by information about the interaction between hypertension and alcohol, but the power of that effect will depend on other factors, such as work schedules, sports seasons, and choices made by friends. Later in this chapter, we will use the CAS lens to explore improvement not from a self-care standpoint but within a microsystem on a hospital unit.

So why is understanding the complexity of systems important for making changes in a health care setting? Complexity theory shifts our thinking from systems as a mechanical, linear interaction to a nonlinear, emergent, and embedded set of interconnected, adaptable elements. There will be times when a health care organization (for example, private-practice office, unit in a hospital, nursing department) will want to "install," "implement," or "roll out" a new process. These words should be concerning because they signal an assumption that change is mechanical. We pull a lever (have training, send a memo), "install" a change, and the system is better. When we hear these words from those who intend to make changes in health care, we need to be wary of their underlying assumptions about the system. Even a basic understanding of the theory and principles of CASs will guide a more realistic (and probably more successful) effort to create change, taking into account the properties that are inherent in the system.

Managing Changes to a System

Now that you have an understanding of how systems respond to change, how do you start managing these changes? There are multiple theories of making change; in fact, entire books have been written on managing change in organizations. Here we present a scenario about reducing falls and injuries due to falls on a hospital unit. We use this scenario to describe the basic elements of change theory, introduce one technique to identify possible changes based on the process diagram, and discuss the PDSA methodology.

Yinzhi Chen, a registered nurse who also holds a doctoral degree, has been the chief nursing officer at the academic Bayside Medical Center (BMC) for the past three years. She is frequently amazed at the size and complexity of BMC. In addition to undergraduate nursing, nurse practitioner, and nurse anesthetist students who fall under her responsibility, there are resident physicians, medical students, pharmacy students and interns, and students from respiratory, physical, and occupational therapy. The educational focus of BMC makes it an exciting (and challenging) organization at which to work.

Today Yinzhi is not focused on the teaching mission but is instead consumed by some rather troubling information. The patient fall rate at BMC has been high and steady for several years. Yinzhi spent many years as a medical/surgical nurse, and she knows that a patient fall can cause serious injury to the patient and is a portent of adverse outcomes for that patient. A patient who falls and has a serious injury such as a hip fracture can have a one-year mortality rate near 33%.[5] As the chief nursing officer, she realizes that there is no simple solution. She'll need to enlist a team of individuals from many professions to solve this problem. She reviews the data from different units and ponders some possible actions. Perhaps a day-long education event about patients' risk of falling? She could start with the lowest-performing ward; it can only go up. Perhaps she could bring in a consultant team to recommend some changes.

Yinzhi decides to confer with Gerry Rogale, the medical chief of staff. He was surprised to see the high rate of falls on so many of the wards. The medicine ward has the poorest performance in the hospital, but Yinzhi and Gerry decide against starting there. The medicine ward has been under some stress due to the retirement of the long-term chief of medicine two months ago and now having an interim chief in place. The physical medicine and rehabilitation (PM&R) unit might be a possibility. Yinzhi and Gerry have had a good working relationship with this group. The PM&R fall rate is a little below the hospital average, and there are strong leaders in the unit in nursing, medicine, and physical therapy. This is a group that could tackle the problem of patient falls and identify some changes that might work for the entire organization. Yinzhi and Gerry agree that this is a reasonable place to start and decide to charge a team to lower the rate of falls on the BMC PM&R unit.

Intentional and Emergent Changes

In the preceding scenario, Yinzhi initially contemplates widespread "installation" of change through an employee education day, but she quickly realizes that this is unlikely to be effective. Pursuing changes in a way that recognizes the inherent properties of a complex adaptive system increases the chance of lasting improvements.

While Yinzhi's initial thoughts were to push change on the entire system, she and Gerry decide on a plan to start with change on one unit in the hospital. Perhaps there they can create and test approaches that will be helpful on other units.

Intentional change. Change that is planned and championed by the leader of a system is sometimes termed *intentional* change. It is often accompanied by a rational case that is made for the changes. One example is the change that occurs when consultants are hired, one option that Yinzhi considered. Intentional change usually comes from outside the system and occurs after a planning period. Intentional change is sometimes required to create a large shift in the processes and patterns within a clinical unit.

Emergent change. *Emergent* change is the type of change that Yinzhi and Gerry decide to pursue. Emergent change contains no *a priori* implemented plan. Rather, emergent change is an adaptive response of a complex system. For emergent change to occur, it has to be driven from within the system itself. Outsiders and consultants may hinder emergent change.

Constructs to Make Systems Changes

Intentional change and emergent change are constructs to approach making changes in a system. These are not "change rules" to be followed; rather, they provide guidance depending on the needs of the system. In truth, either approach may be effective, provided that it accomplishes the following[6]:

1. **Animates people:** People need to get moving and generate experiments that uncover opportunities for improvement.
2. **Provides direction:** A clear aim is a must.
3. **Encourages updating:** Systems changes do not occur once and then stop. Effective change creates an environment with improved situational awareness and close attention to what is occurring in the system. This is recognized by all agents in the system—not just by the leaders.
4. **Facilitates respectful interaction:** As we saw in Chapter 3, interprofessional teams that are focused on improvement develop trust, trustworthiness, and self-respect. These characteristics develop in parallel and are vital for efficient and effective team functioning.

Patterns of Responses to Change/Innovation

After Yinzhi and Gerry decided to take advantage of the interest in making things better in the ordinary course of a day's work, they focused on facilitating emergent change to reduce falls. Their next decision was where to start. They did not "roll out" a program for the entire hospital but focused on identifying a unit that would be best suited to work on the problem. In his theory of "diffusion of innovation," Everett Rogers developed a classification for considering how change is taken up and disseminated within a system.[6] Choosing the right starting place for change depends on identifying the characteristics of the people and system that will be changed.

DEFINED:
Intentional and Emergent Changes
Change that is planned and championed by the leader of a system is sometimes termed intentional *change.* Emergent *change contains no* a priori *implemented plan.*

Classifying the responders. Rogers identified five different patterns of responses to innovation or change (*see* Figure 8-3 on page 131). The classification of responders is based on these patterns:

- **Group 1—Innovators:** Change often starts with innovators. The innovators are the smallest subgroup and often are the creative and passionate individuals.
- **Group 2—Early adopters:** The next group is the early adopters, who are often respected opinion leaders within the system and are role models for others. As shown in Figure 8-3, early adopters are positioned on the initial upslope of accepting and incorporating a change. These individuals (or the systems in which they work) are willing to try changes and work out the bugs to identify what works and what does not work. Yinzhi and Gerry recognize that the PM&R unit is an early adopter unit. With strong leadership in medicine, nursing, and physical therapy, this unit likely is a good place to try new ideas and work out how best to address the patient falls problem.
- **Group 3—Early majority:** The next type of responders is the early majority, who represent a critical stage for widespread acceptance of a change. This is the group that, when successfully adopting a change, is able to bring the change to the peak rate of acceptance. The early majority considers the pros and cons of the change and will discuss the changes with others to get a feel for the situation. Once the early majority adopts a change, more generalized acceptance likely will follow.
- **Group 4—Late majority:** The fourth innovation responder category is the late majority. Those in this group often require a bit of friendly peer pressure to take up an innovation.
- **Group 5—Laggards:** The laggards are the final group. Although this term may seem pejorative, the laggards perform an important cross-checking role. They may be suspicious of a new idea and often look to the past instead of the future. For laggards, resistance to an innovation is rational because they must be certain that important things they value about the current state of affairs will not be lost in the new way of operating.

These response patterns regarding the diffusion of innovation are not intended to be a series of boxes in which to place individuals, clinical units, or microsystems. In reality, each person has times when he or she is an innovator, part of the early majority, or a laggard. Someone who is an innovator in one instance might be a laggard in another. Similarly, an ambulatory pediatric practice might be an innovator in using new computer technology but a laggard in adopting a new form for documenting patient home instructions. The important message from Figure 8-3 is that the diffusion of change is a process that occurs across a continuum. Simply offering a change and hoping that it will be taken up and spread throughout the system is not an effective strategy. Rogers's observations about the different patterns of response to new ideas can help identify where and with whom to develop and carry out new ideas.

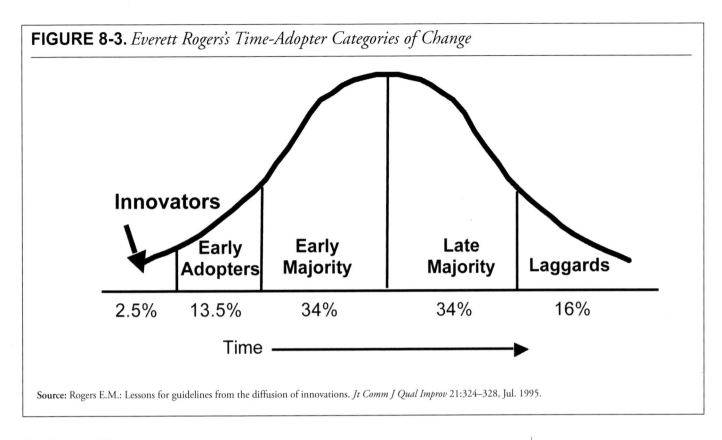

FIGURE 8-3. *Everett Rogers's Time-Adopter Categories of Change*

Source: Rogers E.M.: Lessons for guidelines from the diffusion of innovations. *Jt Comm J Qual Improv* 21:324–328, Jul. 1995.

Barriers to Change

Despite the best planning and targeting of changes, barriers to change are common. Change disrupts the patterns and processes that are in place, so pushback is to be expected. Barriers to change often feel immense and, perhaps, insurmountable. Barriers range from the inertia and comfort of the status quo to process illiteracy and even outcomes ignorance.

Naming the barriers. If barriers to change do not simply melt away, how can we deal with them? We can start by naming a barrier (for example, resistance, apathy) and refrain from naming an individual person. Reactions to changes range from open commitment to public resistance.[1] These reactions may be thought of as stages of readiness for change and may be categorized as follows:

- **Resistance:** Those who openly respond with behaviors and emotions to impede the change display resistance. Resistance is often the "voice" of loss or the "threat" of loss. Exploring what is perceived as loss or a threat can be very revealing and can aid in system redesign.
- **Apathy:** Apathetic individuals show little interest in a change effort.
- **Compliance:** Those who publicly follow the changes but privately disagree with the change are compliant.
- **Commitment:** Those who are fully dedicated to the change demonstrate commitment.

Depending on the change, any one individual may be in any one of these stages. Correctly identifying the stage of readiness for change for key individuals or groups will allow the change team to understand and address the barriers that arise.

Overcoming communication barriers. Communication is the key to building commitment to a change among individuals (*see* Table 8-1 below).[1] Information on why a change is being made and the local historical context for the change decreases anxiety. It is important to anticipate how people will be affected by a change. The early testing cycles of a change should help anticipate what might occur. It is also important to publicize a change, provide clarity about the aim, create excitement about the new opportunities, and show appreciation for everyone's efforts. Note that disparaging those who resist change or those who are apathetic to change is never effective for overcoming barriers. Embracing those who resist or disagree and working to address their concerns demonstrates respect and develops trust while encouraging others to speak up. This approach develops knowledge about the system and may uncover other chances for improvement.

TABLE 8-1.
Techniques That Can Be Helpful When Building Commitment for Change Within a System

Technique	Description and Examples
1. Provide information about the change.	• Recognize the anxiety that comes with change. It is unlikely to be eliminated, but acknowledging it can help. • Share the aim statement of the improvement team. • Show the quality gap (via measures) that exists and which the change(s) is intended to address. • Keep the patient at the center of the change efforts. • Connect the change(s) to the mission and values of the organization.
2. Anticipate how the change will affect people and provide this information to them.	• Be available to answer questions and accept comments. • Always be prepared to study rational objections; someone may have insight that was overlooked by the team. • Share results from tests of change.
3. Gather information from the end users about the resources that will be necessary to make the change.	• Opinion leaders and change agents are helpful, but those who are often in the late majority group or the laggard group (*see* Figure 8-3) also can provide important feedback. • Request formal and visible support from organizational leaders (for example, clinical leaders, nurse unit managers, senior administrators). • Be confident about the process of testing and implementing changes and the desire to make this work with the current system.
4. Publicize the change.	• Tell stories and anecdotes about successful change. • Create a data board in a public space where everyone can follow the progress of the key measures. • Summarize key points and agreements as they are made. • Provide vocal public appreciation for those who are supportive of the change(s).

Source: Adapted from Langley G.J., et. al: *The Improvement Guide: A Practical Approach to Enhancing Organizational Performance.* San Francisco: Jossey-Bass, 1996.

Let's return to the scenario to examine the next steps.

The leaders on the PM&R unit charge an interprofessional team to lead the falls improvement project. The team consists of four members: Jaime Fernandez, one of the floor nurses; Christine Sun, the chief resident in PM&R; Peter Hampton, a physical therapist; and Corinna Ajit, the unit pharmacist. This month, they are joined by Amira Salat, a final-semester nursing student who is interested in PM&R. She is doing a clinical rotation on the ward. The team obtains the patient falls data from Yinzhi. The team members at first don't understand why their unit was chosen to be the first to work on the falls initiative. The data win them over. They are surprised to see that the rate of falls (adjusted for the number of bed-days of care per month) has been stable, with a rather high average, for the past 24 months (see Figure 8-4 on page 134). The rate shows only common cause variation.* If the system on the PM&R unit continues on as is, the unit can expect (or predict) a monthly fall rate between 1.1 (lower control limit) and 12.4 (upper control limit). Because this is a rehabilitation unit that focuses on patient mobility and function, the team is disappointed with these results. The team thought the unit was doing better than this.

Amira is excited to be part of the improvement team while working on the unit. She learned a little about improvement in her earlier courses in nursing school but has not had an opportunity to see a team start from scratch. The PM&R unit team agrees on an aim: "Reduce the fall rate on the BMC PM&R unit by 50% over the next nine months." While the team members are all part of the clinical care process, they recognize the need to have a common process diagram to guide their discussions. Amira agrees to follow a few patients through the care process on the ward and create a deployment flowchart. She shares her efforts with the team at the meeting the following week (see Figure 8-5 on page 134).

Identifying Possible Changes Using Change Concepts

In Chapter 5 we discussed the importance of process literacy. Creating a process model helps develop a common representation of a process and allows a team to identify possible changes to make. The list of possible changes often comes from best practices or from individuals who are part of the process and have ideas about how it can be improved. Whatever it chooses, a team cannot be sure of success until the change is tested and the team evaluates the reaction of the system.

Beyond best practices and personal experience within the system, change concepts can help a team use a process diagram to identify ways to improve the system. *Change concepts* are general principles that can be applied to any clinical process. Langley[1] listed more than 50 change concepts from his work improving many different types of systems. Nelson et al.[8] winnowed down these 50 general change concepts to 10 that are most applicable to health care (*see* Table 8-2 on page 135 and Figure 8-6 on page 136).

---

* See Chapter 7 for information about common cause variation.

FIGURE 8-4. *XmR Control Chart (See Chapter 7) of the Rate of Patient Falls per Bed-Days of Care per Month on the PM&R Unit at Bayside Medical Center**

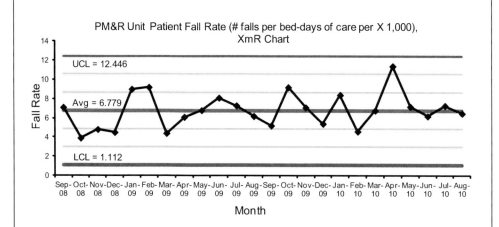

* "Bed-days of care" is the number of days in the month that a hospital bed is occupied by a patient. It is used to normalize the exposure to the risk of falling each month.

FIGURE 8-5. *Deployment Flow Process Diagram of Patient Admission and Fall Assessment on the PM&R Unit at Bayside Medical Center**

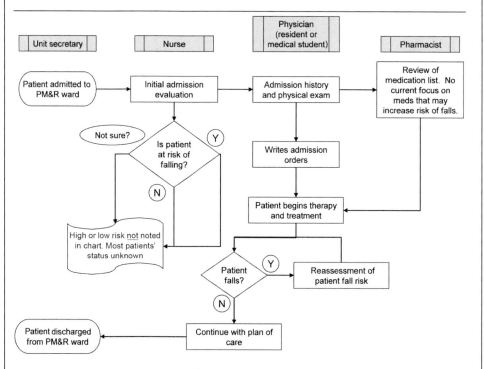

* This is a high-level flow diagram but shows the various people involved in the process. It also demonstrates the lack of a standardized falls risk assessment program and the variable responses to a patient who falls.

A *change concept* "is a general notion or approach to change that has been found to be useful in developing specific ideas for changes that lead to improvement."[1] These generic concepts can clarify a team's thinking about where (and how) in a process change should occur. In some cases, the 10 change concepts merely put names to changes that a team has already identified. If an improvement team has clear and reasonable ideas about where the process needs to change, the change can start there. A team can use the change concepts as a complement to its thinking when it is stalled or when it needs a different approach. The change concepts make a sort of toolbox the team can open when it needs to think differently about the process. For example, change concept 4 in Figure 8-6 is to "eliminate [a] step," and change concept 10 is to "listen to customers (patients, families, staff)." A process flow diagram, like the one shown in Figure 8-6, often identifies unnecessary and repetitive steps in a process;

TABLE 8-2.
Generic Change Concepts for Improving Any Clinical Process

Concept Number	Change Concept Name	Description	Example (*See* Figure 8-6 on Page 136)
1	Modify input	The process has a starting point, and this starting point can be changed.	Screen patients for risk of falling at admission to the unit.
2	Combine steps	The team should combine steps in the process where time and resources can be saved.	Because assessment is completed at admission, falls risk notation ("falling star") is completed up front rather than several days into a patient's admission.
3	Eliminate failures at handoffs	Handoffs require clear, consistent, and reliable transfer of information.	At nursing sign-out, make the falls risk score one of the vital signs.
4	Eliminate a step	The team should identify steps in a process that add no value to the system.	Physical therapists do not need to redo falls assessment. Initial nursing assessment includes adequate information for all professionals.
5	Reorder the sequence of steps	Perhaps prioritizing steps in a different way would help the workflow.	Toileting often occurs after distributing meds. Distributing meds can take a long time, so move toileting to before giving meds.
6	Smooth the workflow in a step	The demand for services causes a large bolus in the number of patients and disrupts the overall flow.	The workup and documentation of possible injuries in a patient who falls is not standardized.
7	Replace with a better value step	Sometimes a step in a process is just not working well and needs to be completely replaced.	Patients are usually randomly assigned to rooms on the ward. Place patients at high risk of falls close to the nurses' station.
8	From knowledge of outcome, redesign process	Outcome and process measures create a powerful impetus for change and can also direct the team to certain specific changes.	Further analysis of the fall rate data shows that patients with a history of stroke have a higher rate of falls.
9	Do tasks in parallel with the main process	Improvements in time and costs can be made by recognition that some tasks can be completed at the same time rather than in sequence.	Falls risk assessment can occur with initial nursing intake.
10	Listen to customers (patients, families, staff)	Input about our processes from the users of our services can often provide significant insight into how to improve what we do.	Families express concern about the use of restraints when patients have acute delirium. Identify alternative ways of preventing falls rather than restraints.

Source: Adapted from Langley G.J., et. al: *The Improvement Guide: A Practical Approach to Enhancing Organizational Performance.* San Francisco: Jossey-Bass, 1996.

FIGURE 8-6. *Example of How 10 Change Concepts Applied to Any Process Can Be Visualized in a Flow Diagram**

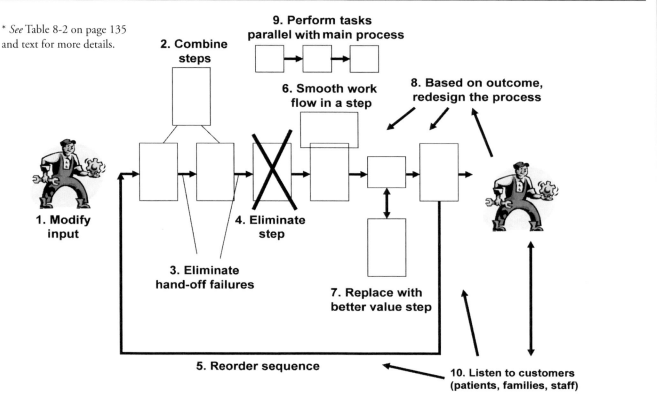

* *See* Table 8-2 on page 135 and text for more details.

2. Combine steps

9. **Perform tasks parallel with main process**

6. **Smooth work flow in a step**

8. **Based on outcome, redesign the process**

1. **Modify input**

4. **Eliminate step**

3. **Eliminate hand-off failures**

7. **Replace with better value step**

5. **Reorder sequence**

10. **Listen to customers (patients, families, staff)**

Source: Adapted from Nelson E.C., Batalden P.B., Lazar J.S. (eds.): *Practice-Based Learning and Improvement: A Clinical Improvement Action Guide,* 2nd ed. Oak Brook, IL: Joint Commission Resources, 2007.

however, it is difficult in a process diagram to identify the opportunity to create changes because a team does not always get feedback from customers. For example, the BMC PM&R unit had been using soft wrist restraints for patients who developed acute delirium while on the unit. While these restraints can be effective for keeping a patient safe for a short period of time, families were troubled by seeing the restraints. This important feedback from families helped the team consider alternatives to restraints to keep patients safe.

Change concepts can help the team brainstorm to create a list of possible changes. Generating this list answers the third question in the model for improvement: What changes can we make that will result in improvement (*see* Figure 8-1)? The team is now ready to try some of these changes.

Amira's work on the process diagram is immensely helpful to the team. The team members immediately recognize that there is no consistent way to identify patients at high risk of falling (see Figure 8-5). Reducing falls is going to be nearly impossible if the team cannot identify the patients who are at high risk. The team decides to test a fall risk assessment tool.

Amira will help Jaime with this tool on the next few patients admitted to the unit. They use the PDSA approach (introduced in Chapter 1) to guide their work (see Figure 8-1):

PDSA 1

Plan—*Jaime will use a standard fall risk assessment tool on the next three patients admitted to him on the PM&R unit.*

Do—*Jaime administered the fall risk assessment tool to Mrs. Perez, a 78-year-old woman who is recovering from a left cerebral stroke; Mr. Browne, a 68-year-old man who had a hip replacement; and Ms. Nichols, a 36-year-old woman who had shoulder surgery. Amira observed each trial and timed the administration of the instrument. Mrs. Perez and Mr. Browne were identified as being at high risk for falling, but Ms. Nichols was not.*

Study—*Jaime and Amira debriefed with the improvement team. Although the fall risk assessment seems to be accurate in that it identified patients at high risk, it was cumbersome to administer. It took Jaime an average of 4 minutes and 23 seconds for each patient. In addition, some of the information on the form is already collected as part of the intake information on the ward.*

Act—*Conducting a fall risk assessment is important, but the current form is too cumbersome to use in addition to completing other duties.*

Amira identifies a short form from the material Peter brought back from the conference. The short form of the fall risk assessment tool works much better than the old form. Jaime found it easy to administer, it provided valuable information, and Amira scored the administration time at just under 40 seconds, which is acceptable to both nurses and patients.

Now that the team members can reliably identify patients at high risk, the team tries several other interventions to decrease the rate of falls. It moves high-risk patients closer to the nurses' station and pilot tests bed alarms and chair alarms. It also identifies each high-risk patient with a "falling star" on his or her doorpost and purchases some low beds for very high-risk patients. Table 8-3 on page 138 provides a complete list of changes the team tried.

After six months of work and 12 different PDSA cycles, the team is pleased to see that the fall rate has dropped below the lower control limit, indicating special cause variation (see Figure 8-7 on page 138). The team is encouraged by this signal in the data that reflects the work done. The unit now has a reliable fall risk assessment and evidence-based interventions that prevent patient falls.

The team meets with Yinzhi and Gerry to discuss its progress. They are excited about the results and are anxious to spread the interventions to other units in the hospital. Figure 8-7 shows the updated XmR chart, with a few months of fall rates under the mean of 6.5 and a special cause represented in the most recent data point. The arrows indicate the changes that were tested. Dark arrows indicate changes that were successful and maintained, and lighter arrows are changes that were not successful and, therefore, not continued.

TABLE 8-3.

List of Changes That Were Tried by the Bayside Medical Center PM&R Unit Improvement Team

- Patient sitters
- Sound monitors
- Moving high-risk patients closer to the nurses' station
- Bed alarms
- Strip alarms
- New cardiac chairs
- Painting walls behind toilet a dark color to add contrast for male patients
- Chairs with arm rests
- Gait belts
- Hip protectors
- Low beds with floor mats
- Red fall precaution bracelets
- Yellow "Falling Stars"
- Electronic option for requesting fall consults
- Trial of new slipper socks with rubber soles

FIGURE 8-7. *Updated and Annotated XmR Chart of the Falls Rate for the PM&R Unit at Bayside Medical Center**

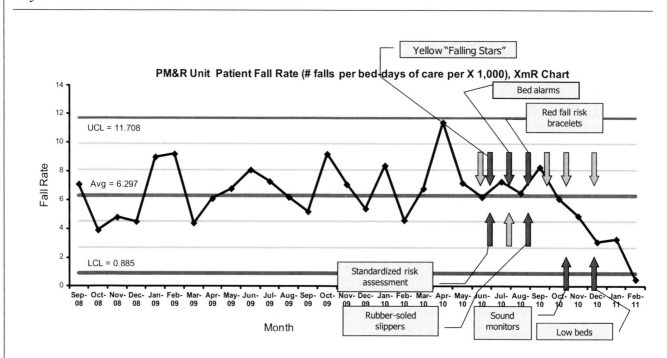

* Arrows indicate changes to the process. Dark arrows = successful changes; light arrows = unsuccessful changes.

Using the PDSA Methodology to Test and Assess Changes

As introduced in Chapter 1, the PDSA methodology is used to test changes in a system (*see* Figure 8-8 on page 140). PDSA is intended to test small changes, but sometimes it is applied to large-scale changes or to planned changes that have not been completed. For example, a hospital might state that the implementation of a new electronic medical record (EMR) is being done using PDSA methodology in the following way:

Plan—Implement a new EMR.

Do—Get the new EMR installed.

Study—Assess the uptake and use of the new EMR.

Act—Improve the use of the new EMR, based on preliminary findings.

This example demonstrates a common misconception and misuse of PDSA. PDSA is best used when applied to testing small changes in a system. It is generally not appropriate for testing the rollout of a new massive change effort. It is not intended to guide the implementation of a large-scale program. It is intended to test one change with a few patients in one setting on a small scale. This may seem too small to make a difference, but the goal is to build information step-by-step. The improvement team should not stop at just one PDSA cycle. Jaime and Amira performed the first PDSA cycle for the BMC PM&R falls team by trying an assessment tool on three patients. This test provided a wealth of information for the team. The team recognized that the tool was effective but cumbersome to administer. If falls assessment was to become a routine part of the admission process, a faster, more reliable form would be needed. The four phases of the PDSA cycle are as follows (*see* Figure 8-8):

- **Plan phase:** The team starts in the plan phase, where the goal of the test of change is stated. This is different from the overall aim of the improvement project (as discussed in Chapter 4) because these plans are very focused and directed at the immediate test of change. The plan phase also encourages the team to create a hypothesis about what will happen when this change is tried. Finally, the plan phase specifies who will do what and where and when this will occur.

- **Do phase:** Carrying out the test and documenting observations about the test occurs in the do phase. The evaluation of the do phase may be quantitative, but often with small tests of change, a qualitative analysis is equally effective to determine what occurred.

- **Study phase:** The study phase is where a complete analysis of the data is done. The outcome is compared to the predicted outcome, and the outcome is summarized.

- **Act phase:** The act phase consists of determining the consequences of the change. What will be the objective for the next PDSA cycle? The act phase from one PDSA cycle flows into the plan phase of the subsequent cycle.

FIGURE 8-8. *The Plan–Do–Study–Act (PDSA) Methodology for Testing Small Changes in a System*

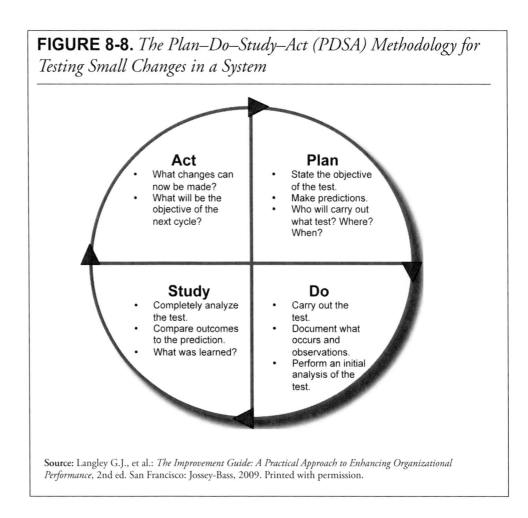

Source: Langley G.J., et al.: *The Improvement Guide: A Practical Approach to Enhancing Organizational Performance*, 2nd ed. San Francisco: Jossey-Bass, 2009. Printed with permission.

Assessing successive PDSA cycles. PDSA cycles are iterative and build on one another. Figure 8-9 on page 141 shows an example of successive PDSA cycles progressing "uphill" as the improvement in the system increases over time. Each PDSA cycle generates new knowledge about the system as tests are tried. Each successive PDSA cycle requires an increase in complexity as knowledge about the system grows. It is never intended that one PDSA cycle will achieve the aim that is stated at the outset. Rather, each PDSA cycle is a small experiment that advances the team's knowledge about the system. Recall that systems behave in complex, adaptive ways, and it is difficult to predict how the system will respond. Each PDSA cycle allows the team to assess how the system responds to the change that is made. The changes that are successful are maintained and amplified, and those that are not successful are discarded. The falls team kept a running total of the changes that were tried and which were maintained and which were discontinued.

Monitoring and tracking PDSA cycles. The most successful users of PDSA are those who monitor and track the cycles in an organized fashion. This is akin to maintaining a lab notebook in laboratory research. As the PDSA cycles grow in number, the team may forget what Cycles 1, 2, and 3 contained because each cycle grows on the previous

FIGURE 8-9. *Successive PDSA Cycles over Time* *

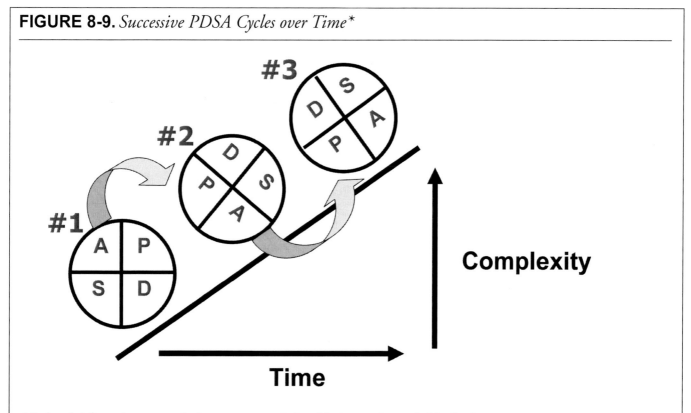

* Each cycle informs the next one. As time goes on, complexity of the interventions and trials often increases.

Source: Adapted from Nelson E.C., Batalden P.B., Lazar J.S. (eds.): *Practice-Based Learning and Improvement: A Clinical Improvement Action Guide*, 2nd ed. Oak Brook, IL: Joint Commission Resources, 2007.

one. By the time the team gets to Cycle 15 (or 23 or 37), it may not recall what occurred in the early cycles. Having a lab notebook to keep track of the tests of change is a convenient way to monitor the changes that have been tried.

Embedding knowledge gained from PDSA cycles into a system. After a team has identified and studied effective interventions in a system with rapid-cycle PDSA methodology, how can these changes be embedded in a system? What is to prevent these good practices that improved outcomes from decaying over time? Sustaining changes in a system requires at least two elements: (1) interventions that are hardwired into the system and (2) regular review of process and outcome measures. Both require the attention of leaders (*see* Chapter 9 for more on sustaining change). In this chapter's example, Amira and Jaime implemented a tool through several PDSA cycles for fall risk stratification of new admissions. Making this a lasting part of the work on the PM&R unit will require that the new form be integrated into the admission routine for all nurses. Knowledge of the usual process of admission (*see* Figure 8-5) will help, as will support from the leadership on the unit. Without the regular evaluation of measures (*see* Figure 8-7), the lasting effectiveness and sustainability of the change will be nearly impossible to assess. PDSA cycles encourage rigor and also demand humility from the improvement team. The rigor comes from the discipline of using a standard, focused methodology for making change that requires iterative hypothesis generation coupled with measurement of outcomes. The humility comes with the recognition and realization that complex systems react in often unpredictable, adaptive ways. With hypothesis generation, careful measurement, and synthesis of outcomes, a team can determine whether the changes it tries truly lead to improvements.

Summary

Managing change requires planning, practice, and patience. A system will not adopt a change simply because you are the clinical leader; rather, successful change in complex systems is often the cumulative effect of many small changes over time. Research studies that use elegant statistical analyses such as linear regression often identify the individual factors that have the most influence on outcomes. When this information is applied to a local setting, it is only as good as the understanding of the local culture and context. No research, no matter how closely it resembles the local setting, will be seamlessly translated to your setting. The complex adaptive nature of a system does not allow this simple implementation. Those who profess a simple translation are often assuming a simple linear relationship between intervention and outcome, but such simple relationships rarely occur.

To improve the rate of patient falls at Bayside Medical Center, Yinzhi and Gerry used principles from complex adaptive systems and Rogers's diffusion of innovation theory. They chose a unit with strong opinion leaders and gave them the support they needed (including data) to identify and test a series of changes over time. The PM&R unit team tested changes representing a wide variety of change concepts. The team learned which changes worked in its setting by tracking the results over time. The success and lessons learned on that unit can be spread to others at BMC. As team members said, "If they can do it, so can we" and "Oh, I see how that can work." However, as Chapter 9 describes, this won't happen automatically.

Managing change is a systematic process that entails the use of evidence-based approaches as well as artful responses to local conditions. Testing and assessing build knowledge about a system in a rigorous and systematic way that helps to generate a more reliable system. Change is not easy, but when it is done well, it is immensely satisfying because the team is able to make system-level changes to improve processes and outcomes for patients.

References

1. Langley G.J., et. al: *The Improvement Guide: A Practical Approach to Enhancing Organizational Performance.* San Francisco: Jossey-Bass, 1996.
2. Institute for Healthcare Improvement: *Knowledge Center.* http://www.ihi.org/knowledge (accessed Oct. 28, 2011).
3. Batalden P.B., Davidoff F.: What is "quality improvement" and how can it transform health care? *Qual Saf Health Care* 16:2–3, Feb. 2007.
4. Plsek P.: Redesigning health care with insights from the science of complex adaptive systems. In Committee on Quality of Health Care in America, Institute of Medicine: *Crossing the Quality Chasm: A New Health System for the 21st Century.* Washington, DC: National Academy Press, 2001.
5. Swift C.G.: Care of older people: Falls in late life and their consequences—Implementing effective services. *BMJ* 322:855–857, Apr. 2001.
6. Weick K.E.: Emergent change as a universal in organizations. In Beer M., Nohria N. (eds.): *Breaking the Code of Change.* Boston: Harvard Business School Press, 2000, pp. 223–242.
7. Rogers E.M.: Lessons for guidelines from the diffusion of innovations. *Jt Comm J Qual Improv* 21:324–328, Jul. 1995.
8. Nelson E.C., Batalden P.B., Lazar J.S. (eds.): *Practice-Based Learning and Improvement: A Clinical Improvement Action Guide*, 2nd ed. Oak Brook, IL: Joint Commission Resources, 2007.

CHAPTER 9

Spreading Improvements

OBJECTIVES

After reading this chapter, you will be able to do the following:

1. Identify effective strategies for sustaining and spreading change.
2. Follow a step-by-step approach to planning spread efforts.
3. Avoid common mistakes and plan for success.

An improvement team in a teaching hospital is very excited about improvements it has made in using Teach Back with patients throughout the hospital stay to assess patients' and family caregivers' understanding of discharge instructions and ability to perform self-care. Teach Back is a method of interacting with patients to confirm that the health care provider has explained what the patient needs to know in a way that the patient understands. A patient's understanding is confirmed when he or she explains what's been said back to the health care provider.[1] It is one of the methods used to reduce the likelihood of patients returning to the hospital unnecessarily after discharge because they did not fully understand how to take care of themselves after they returned home (or because their family caregivers did not know how to administer care).[2]

The improvement team, led by nurse educator Faiza Okoye, also includes a staff nurse, a hospitalist (that is, a hospital-based physician), a pharmacist, a resident, and a nursing assistant from a selected medical/surgical unit. This inpatient team is also part of a larger cross-continuum team that's been working to reduce unnecessary readmissions to the hospital. (The cross-continuum team comprises representatives from the hospital's community partners, including a local nursing home, a home health agency, and a large primary care practice affiliated with the hospital.) When interviewing patients, the inpatient improvement team quickly learned that one of the issues contributing to readmissions was that patients were often confused about which medications to take when they returned home.

Faiza suggested that they use the Teach Back method to help patients better understand their discharge instructions. They began by watching a Teach Back video[3] and trying the method with one or two patients. Under the guidance of the nurse educator, they observed each other and learned how to interact with the patients in a more effective way. They studied how often patients could explain back what they had reviewed with them and improved their Teach Back skills. Faiza then worked with all the nurses, residents, and nursing assistants on the unit so that all staff members who interacted with patients were confident in their use of Teach Back. They were so enthusiastic about the patients' response and their own experience that they wanted to share this new method with care teams on other units.

They presented their work to the cross-continuum team. The executive sponsor of the cross-continuum team assigned the chief nursing officer and the director of the residency program to be the spread leaders for Teach Back. The spread leaders, together with Faiza, nursing managers, residents, and the improvement team, developed a spread plan for the hospital that included the following components:

- *The leaders and the improvement team made presentations at medical staff, residency program, and unit meetings.*
- *The nurse educator developed a training schedule for units that were being introduced to Teach Back, first training one or two nurses and residents who could become (with the support of the nurse managers on these units and the residency director) the mentors on the new units.*
- *As the mentors became capable of supporting the new units, the next five units were scheduled for training by the nurse educator.*
- *Data on the effectiveness of the Teach Back method were collected in each unit (such as the percentage of patients who could teach back at least 75% of the information they received).*
- *Teach Back continued to be an agenda item at medical staff, residency program, and nursing unit meetings to reinforce its importance and to share learning about its use.*
- *To ensure continued use of Teach Back, it was incorporated into the yearly competency training for nurses and medical assistants, as well as into the residency training program.*
- *Nursing, pharmacy, and medical students who spent time learning on the units were also given training so they could contribute to the Teach Back efforts.*

The cross-continuum team received regular updates on the readmission rates and on the spread of Teach Back within the hospital. Members of the cross-continuum team from community partners (nursing homes, home health agencies, area offices on aging, and so on) saw the potential for using Teach Back in their facilities and programs. With coaching from the spread leaders and Faiza, the nurse educator, they developed a plan for bringing Teach Back to their staff so that the patient education could be reinforced and strengthened once the patients were discharged.

Spread: Overview and Definition

Spread is defined as the process by which new ideas are communicated over time through a social system,[4] with the intended outcome being the adoption of the new ideas. Spread is part of an overall process of improvement—a process that involves first testing and refining new ideas or processes on a small scale, such as in a single medical/surgical unit in a hospital or one primary care clinic, and then ensuring that the new processes are embedded in the daily work of the clinicians and staff in those initial units (that is, ensuring that they are implemented). After the improvements have been implemented in the initial units, they are ready for broader adoption across the organization and/or to other organizations. The preceding vignette describes the adoption of the Teach Back method developed in one unit by others within the hospital.

Spread sometimes occurs without much intervention, but this natural diffusion of innovation may take a long time to complete, as in the now-famous description by Everett Rogers of the spread of a new type of seed corn—where the benefits alone were not enough to promote rapid spread of its use.[4] Those involved in making care safer and better for patients want to accelerate change so that it occurs as quickly as possible, because a delay in the adoption of better ideas and processes means the potential for patient harm or the delivery of less-than-optimal care. In this chapter, the term *spread* refers to a planned approach that includes the methods leaders can use to strategically plan and execute a system that accelerates the adoption of new ideas or processes as the scope—or scale—of the change expands and to ensure that the new ideas are sustained over time.[5]

The example we will use to illustrate a successful approach to spread is a hand hygiene initiative carried out at Iowa Health Des Moines (IHDM) to decrease infections and improve patient safety.[6] The hand hygiene initiative initially involved the three hospitals that are part of IHDM: Iowa Methodist Medical Center, Blank Children's Hospital, and Iowa Lutheran Hospital. The case study in this chapter describes the initial spread processes at IHDM, which was able to achieve and sustain a 90% rate of adoption of prescribed hand hygiene policies by January 2009, as compared with a 60% rate at the start of the initiative in April 2008 (*see* Figure 9-1 on page 148).[7]

The steps in the approach include the following:
>Step 1—Setting a Foundation for Spread
>Step 2—Developing an Initial Plan for Spread
>Step 3—Carrying Out and Refining the Spread Plan

Step 1: Setting a Foundation for Spread

One of the biggest mistakes that leaders make with spread initiatives is to not plan early enough for how they will spread an improvement that is developed in a pilot site. While it is often said that in order to spread, one needs something to spread, it is also the case that spread does not happen without planning and preparation. There are several recommended steps to consider in establishing a solid foundation for spread,[5] including establishing a team to lead the spread effort and ensuring alignment between the strategic goals of the organization and the spread effort. It is important to note

> **DEFINED: Spread**
>
> Spread *is the process by which new ideas are communicated over time through a social system, with the intended outcome being the adoption of the new ideas.*

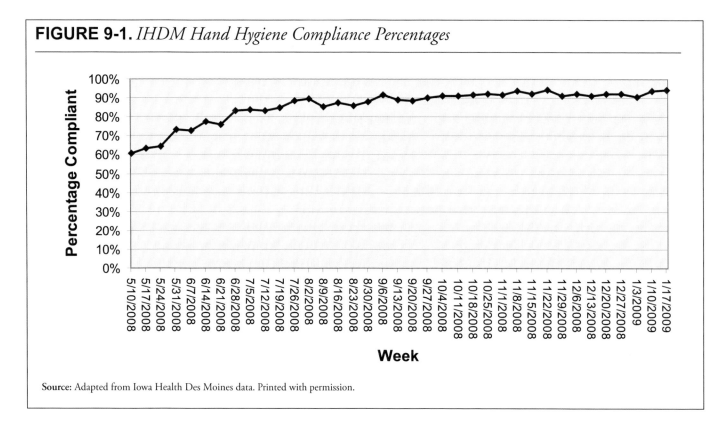

FIGURE 9-1. *IHDM Hand Hygiene Compliance Percentages*

Source: Adapted from Iowa Health Des Moines data. Printed with permission.

here that the primary responsibility for planning and organizing spread rests with the leadership of the organization or system. Frontline staff play an important role in spread; they are members of teams where the improvements are tested and refined so that they can be easily shared with others. The support structure needed to actually spread changes across a system must be established, supported, and maintained by the leadership.

Establishing a Spread Team

A *spread team* is a group established by an organization's leaders to guide and monitor a spread effort. The senior leaders at IHDM established an interprofessional team to identify and carry out improvements in the system's hand hygiene processes. The team included the following members:

- **Team sponsors:** The executive director of women's services and the director of clinical quality provided resources, support, and encouragement to the IHDM team.
- **Day-to-day leader:** The person responsible for the day-to-day activities of the team was an infection prevention nurse at IHDM. This person who functioned as the spread team leader convened team meetings, helped the team make and carry out its plans, kept track of tests that were under way, ensured that the data needed to support the team's work were collected and displayed, and provided update reports to senior leaders.
- **Facilitator:** The quality improvement coordinator helped to ensure that team meetings were well organized and productive and that all members of the team

---

DEFINED: Spread Team

A spread team *is a group established by an organization's leaders to guide and monitor a spread effort.*

contributed to its work and progress. The coordinator also assisted the leader in keeping track of tests, data, and reports.

- **Physician leaders:** Two physician leaders (the hospital epidemiologist and the vice president of medical affairs) promoted the initiative among physicians during medical staff meetings and followed up personally with other physician leaders and individual physicians, as needed, throughout the initiative.
- **Other clinicians and staff:** Members included clinicians and staff members who were involved in initially identifying, testing, and refining changes to improve hand washing in the initial units as well as representatives from the target units in each hospital. They included nurse supervisors and managers from medical and surgical services, oncology, rehabilitation, critical care, behavioral health, the emergency department, a resident, and representatives from marketing, epidemiology, and environmental services.

Aligning a Spread Effort with Strategic Goals

For spread to be successful, leadership needs to provide a clear and unambiguous message that the status quo is unacceptable and that the improvements to be spread are central to the future success of the organization. Since 2000, when the chief medical officer established a corporate clinical performance improvement (CPI) department responsible for quality performance and clinical safety improvement across the system, IHDM has dedicated itself to improving patient safety.[7]

Before the IHDM hand hygiene initiative was begun, The Joint Commission noted lapses in hand hygiene during a resurvey. This got the attention of the system's leaders. The chief executive officer, other members of the executive team, and managers across IHDM sent a clear message through written and verbal communication channels that hand hygiene was a priority for the organization and that process changes should be developed and spread across IHDM. To emphasize the importance of this effort, hospital leaders visited units and departments to listen to and encourage staff as the changes in the hand hygiene process were initiated and spread.

Establishing a Spread Aim

A *spread aim* is a clear, concise statement of what an organization intends to accomplish. A good spread aim should address what is being spread, the target audience or population, the time frame, and the expected level of improvement—essentially, the "what," "who," "when," and "how much" of spread. In April 2008 the spread team at IHDM developed an aim statement: "Iowa Health–Des Moines employees will demonstrate 90% compliance with hand hygiene opportunities by August 1, 2008. Executive directors and managers will be sent weekly reports on hand hygiene compliance in their areas and will follow up with employees. They will send a clear message that hand hygiene is a top priority for patient care at IHDM."

The expectations for hand hygiene were clearly spelled out in a hand hygiene policy that had originally been developed several years earlier and then revised prior to

> **DEFINED: Spread Aim**
> *A* spread aim *is a clear, concise statement of what an organization intends to accomplish.*

the launch of the hand hygiene spread effort. The policy was used as the basis for determining compliance for the spread aim.

Step 2: Developing an Initial Plan for Spread

The spread plan addresses the question of *how* the organization will reach the goals outlined in the spread aim. There are a number of methods that can be used to organize spread activities, including everything from large-scale campaigns (for example, the Institute for Healthcare Improvement's 100,000 Lives Campaign and 5 Million Lives Campaign) to the use of extension agents working locally.[8] The appropriate method depends on the level of resources (time and money), the characteristics of the organizational structure (such as centralized or decentralized), and the expected reception of the new ideas (resistant, skeptical, and so on).

Spread plan elements. While the methods for spread may differ, there are elements that are common among them that must be included in any successful spread effort:
- A communication system to share information and resources
- A way to connect the people to maximize learning and support
- A measurement system to track progress and results
- A process for making adjustments in the spread plan, as needed

Leaders at IHDM utilized an already established process for chartering teams (for example, the hand hygiene team) to develop solutions to quality and safety problems and then spread them across their system, using the facility, department, and unit structure to imbed the new practices. They called the effort the One Touch Campaign, as a way to generate interest and energy and to emphasize its importance.

The spread team at IHDM went out and asked those at the bedside and in the ancillary areas at each hospital what beliefs they had about hand hygiene and what they perceived as barriers to cleaning their hands. They found two important factors that were contributing to less-than-optimal hand washing:
- The gel containers weren't being refilled promptly and/or they weren't being used because the gel created skin problems for staff.
- Many staff and clinicians believed that using gloves took the place of cleaning hands, not understanding that putting gloves on with unwashed hands would leave germs on the outside of the gloves and pose a risk to patients.

To address these issues, the spread team worked with the distributor to replace gel with foam and installed 1,800 new foam container holders (which IHDM received for free from the manufacturer), including one in and one outside every room to ensure that they were conveniently located. Even though mounting that many new container holders in more convenient locations was challenging, staff were able to complete the work in three weeks, reflecting the priority of the campaign for the hospitals. The spread team also addressed the misperception about using gloves through an educational program that was part of the team's larger communication plan (described in the following section).

Developing a Communication Plan

A good communication plan is needed for any spread effort in order to fulfill two primary purposes: (1) build awareness of the new ideas and (2) provide technical knowledge and support to those ready to adopt the ideas. The purposes should be matched with the appropriate methods of communication.[9] For example, large meetings may help to build awareness, while one-to-one conversations may be more effective for moving people closer to the decision to adopt or to provide details about how to make the improvements.

The communication plan that the spread team used did the following:

- It built awareness by holding a systemwide kickoff event and developing and displaying 1,000 posters in prominent locations throughout the hospitals (including on each unit).
- It provided technical knowledge about correct hand-washing techniques and principles through online educational modules (which included signing a hand hygiene pledge) that all staff were required to complete.
- It incorporated a hand hygiene policy into the curriculum for the spread effort. In addition, the infection prevention and control nurse leader and hospital epidemiologist worked directly with the residents on infection prevention and control, emphasizing hand hygiene. The educational curriculum also addressed two other important aspects of communication: making the case for why a change is important and simplifying the steps needed to adopt the change. The training emphasized the importance of correct hand hygiene techniques, including why it's important to clean one's hands before putting on gloves and how the foam containers were changed to make it easier for staff to follow the hand hygiene policy.

Addressing response to change. Smart communication strategies address how potential adopters will view the new way of doing things. Rogers[4] identified five characteristics of an innovation that can contribute to the rate of adoption of a new idea or process. The characteristics include the perceived relative advantage of the change; the complexity of the change; its compatibility with the culture, values, and structures currently in place; how observable the new process is to potential adopters; and whether adopters can try the process before committing to its implementation. Through its communication methods and messages, the spread team presented the hand hygiene techniques as practices that would result in fewer infections for patients, as something relatively simple and easy to do (for example, the foam container holders were placed conveniently in and near patient rooms), and as easily observable to both staff and patients. After the policy was established, the spread team continued to gather information as staff took steps to follow the policy and incorporate its practices into daily workflows (that is, making the change "trialable").

Using the Social System for Spread

The social system for spread includes the individuals and groups in the target population—that is, the locations where the transition from the old system to the

Large meetings may help to build awareness, while one-to-one conversations may be more effective for moving people closer to the decision to adopt or to provide details about how to make the improvements.

new one takes place. Spread is successful when a new idea or process is adopted by the members of the social system in the target population. However, because individuals in a social system do not necessary adopt changes at the same time (as Rogers identified and as described in Chapter 8), moving new ideas from a successful site to the target population is not always a simple process.

The spread team at IHDM had two strategies to maximize relationships in the social system at IHDM to accelerate spread: (1) using the department and unit structure and (2) removing environmental barriers.

Using the department and unit structure. The IHDM spread team used the organization's department and unit structure to reach all staff and clinicians, including nurses, physicians, residents, environmental services, ancillary services, and the emergency department. Each nurse manager was put in charge of his or her unit's performance, ensuring that nurses and all staff members were aware of and followed the hand-washing policies. In addition, physician leaders played an important role in communicating with other physicians. For example, when the head of a major ancillary department was made aware of the data in his department, he immediately reinforced the new processes with his physicians. Also, the resident on the spread team served as a liaison between the spread team, the residents, and the physicians. All staff were encouraged not only to clean their own hands but also to give feedback to any physicians, nurses, or residents who were not following the hand hygiene process. Clinical faculty also communicated and reinforced the hand-washing policies with the residents.

Removing environmental barriers. As discussed earlier, the spread team at IHDM identified an environmental and structural issue: the installation of new foam containers. Such structural issues, or transition issues, can slow individuals' willingness to adopt new ideas.[10] Installing functional containers at appropriate sites removed some barriers. Other examples of such obstacles include features of the information system, staffing policies or procedures, and compensation or reimbursement systems. It is the responsibility of the spread leaders to "listen" to the target population to understand barriers to adoption and develop ways to overcome them.[11]

Measurement

A measurement system for spread includes the main outcome measures of the process or system of interest and the rate of spread of the specific improvements. In addition to the measurement system, a feedback system is needed to provide information on progress in reaching the organization's spread goals to the executive leadership, the spread team, and the adopters in the target population.

Collecting the data. The spread team at IHDM developed a hand hygiene monitoring tool and then took it to various areas of the hospitals to get feedback. The team revised the tool based on that feedback and selected monitors on each of the units. In each of the three hospitals, a manager on each unit and ancillary unit chose someone to do the monitoring—someone who really believed in what hand hygiene can do for infection rates. Each monitor received education on how to collect the data and complete the observations. To reduce the burden of data collection and reporting, the monitors counted 10 "before-patient contact" and 10 "after-patient contact" opportunities each week and entered their data using an online survey tool. From those data, results for each unit were sent in the form of weekly reports to all units. Also included in the weekly report were job codes across the board—from physicians to nursing and all ancillary staff—so that reports showed the performance of physicians, nurses, residents, and other staff by job category.

Sharing the data. The data were prominently displayed and discussed in each unit. If the data indicated a lack of compliance with the hand hygiene policy, the unit manager, department director, or physician leader would follow up with members of the unit or department.

Accountability for the data. Units were held accountable for anyone who visited their unit—not just their own staff. So if someone was on a unit, he or she counted in the observations for that unit. This created an environment of accountability in the units so that unit staff felt responsible for what went on in their own units.

Responding to the data. At the same time that the data were being shared openly, the message was also being sent that the data were being used for improvement rather than for judgment. The spread team purposely asked hospital leadership not to impose punitive measures on staff who didn't clean their hands. Leaders approached the campaign as a collaborative effort with staff, viewing it as an opportunity for employee growth and enhanced competence.

At the same time that the data were being shared openly, the message was also being sent that the data were being used for improvement rather than for judgment.

Because the focus of the campaign was on hand hygiene, the measure of interest (in this case, the outcome measure) that was tracked was compliance with the hand hygiene policy for all three hospitals combined—with a goal of 90%. The process measure was the completion of 10 "before-" and "after-" patient contact opportunities by the monitors, with a goal of 100% of the monitoring counts being completed. An additional measure the spread team used to ensure that staff were not suffering adverse skin effects from the hand washing and cleansing was the skin conditions of staff hands, as reported on two staff surveys over a period of a year.

Positive reinforcement was an important part of the campaign as well. The units that had met the goal of 90% were highlighted in the weekly e-mails, and their data were attached. Unit celebrations and other events were held to recognize achievement and to build energy and enthusiasm. For example, to add some fun to the campaign, two nurse managers dressed as clowns visited top-performing units with a wagon full of candy. System leaders also got involved in the celebration. The chief operations officer and another administrator rounded in a "hand" costume, complimenting people cleaning their hands as they made their rounds.

After a period of eight months, the spread team and hospital leaders started highlighting the units that were not meeting hand hygiene compliance in the weekly e-mail. To sustain the improvements (and to ensure that the hand hygiene policy was embedded in unit and department processes and culture), the spread team continued to do weekly measurement of hand hygiene for a year. Then, for four months, the team switched to collecting the data every two weeks. Following that, the team collected data monthly for six months. It is now collecting and publishing data every quarter.

Step 3: Carrying Out and Refining the Spread Plan

It is the responsibility of the spread team to gather information about the spread process as it unfolds in the organization. The spread team plays an important role in monitoring the process and recommending adjustments, as needed, to ensure that the spread goals are met. Communication plans, materials and information, support and mentorship, infrastructure issues, and social system issues all may need attention during a spread effort.

To gather information about how the campaign was progressing, the leaders of the IHDM spread team visited the units, identifying issues with the monitoring process and barriers that surfaced. For example, the spread leaders followed up with unit managers and physician leaders when the data indicated either a lack of awareness or other issues contributing to low monitoring scores.

Sustaining Improvement

Part of the work of refining and strengthening the spread plan involves taking action to ensure that the changes made during a spread effort are sustained over time. IHDM built a number of actions into its campaign that contributed to the high level of hand hygiene IHDM was able to sustain over time, including the following:

- It established and documented standard processes in the hand hygiene policy.
- It set the expectation that hand hygiene is a standard part of every staff member's and clinician's daily responsibilities.
- It used ongoing monitoring, data collection, and reporting to keep the focus on following the policy.
- It developed an online educational module to ensure that all current and new staff would have a solid foundation in the hand hygiene policy.
- It assigned ownership initially through the spread team; after a year and a half, responsibility for monitoring and follow-up was transferred to operational and managerial leaders.
- It addressed the social aspects of change by using positive reinforcement, incorporated a fun culture into the campaign, and celebrated and recognized high-performing units and departments.

Summary

The experience of IHDM in launching and supporting a successful spread effort to improve hand hygiene illustrates a number of key features that can help an organization achieve its goals and sustain improvement over time. While planning and leading spread efforts is the responsibility of an organization's leaders, staff, clinicians, and even trainees play important roles in testing, refining, and helping others to understand and adopt new ideas and processes. In fact, learners can contribute substantially to the spread of improvement through grassroots efforts like those of the Institute for Healthcare Improvement Open School to spread the use of the WHO surgical checklist.[12]

Recommended Spread Effort Components

The following are recommended components for leaders to consider in planning and carrying out successful spread efforts:

- Agenda setting and active involvement of leaders, including a designated spread team
- A clear aim, with measurable targets and a time line
- A spread plan that includes a set of ideas or practices, a way to attract and support adopters, thoughtful use of the social system and attention to structural issues, a measurement and feedback system, and a method to refine the plan, as needed
- Hard wiring of new practices into established policies and procedures, monitoring and tracking of results over time, and attention to cultural issues so that staff, providers, and trainees continue to learn, grow, and feel connected to the ongoing improvements over time

A Framework for Spread[8] (*see* Figure 9-2 on page 156) provides more detail about these components and serves as a guide for leaders to use in incorporating the following into their spread strategy: the role of leadership, the organizational setup to support spread, the description of the new ideas, methods of communication, nurturing of the social system, measurement and feedback systems, and knowledge management. The framework is not prescriptive. Rather, it suggests some general areas for an organization or a team to consider as it undertakes a spread project. Through effective spread, improvements are shared and adopted more broadly, contributing to improved performance by the organization or system and ultimately to health care improvement.

FIGURE 9-2. *A Framework for Spread*

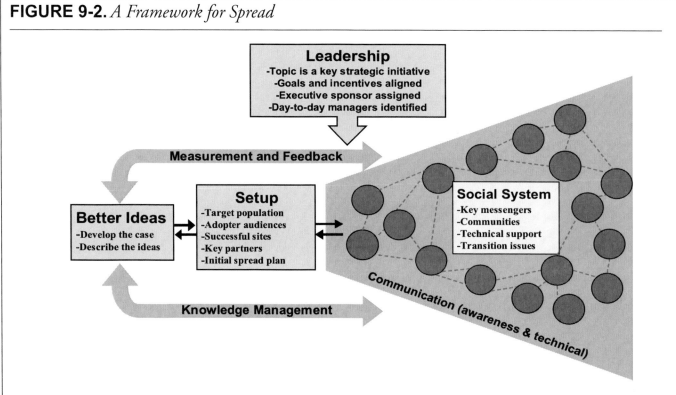

Source: Nolan K., et al.: Using a framework for spread: The case of patient access in the Veterans Health Administration. *Jt Comm J Qual Improv* 31:339–347, 2005.

References

1. DeWalt D.A., et al.: *Health Literacy Universal Precautions Toolkit.* (AHRQ Publication No. 10-0046-EF). Rockville, MD: Agency for Healthcare Research and Quality, Apr. 2010.

2. Schillinger D., et al.: Closing the loop: Physician communication with diabetic patients who have low health literacy. *Arch Intern Med* 163:83–90, Jan. 13, 2003.

3. American Medical Association Health Literacy Program: *Health Literacy Video.* http://www.ama-assn.org/ama/pub/about-ama/ama-foundation/our-programs/public-health/health-literacy-program/health-literacy-video-page (accessed Oct. 18, 2011.)

4. Rogers E.: *Diffusion of Innovations.* New York: The Free Press, 1995.

5. Nolan K.M., Schall M.W.: A framework for spread. In Schall M.W., Nolan K.M. (eds.): *Spreading Improvement Across Your Health Care Organization.* Oak Brook, IL: Joint Commission Resources and the Institute for Healthcare Improvement, 2007, pp.1–24.

6. Personal communication between the author and Pat Busick, M.S., C.I.A., Iowa Lutheran Hospital, and Julie Gibbons, R.N., B.S.N., C.I.C., Iowa Health Des Moines, Feb. 18, 2011.

7. Nolan K., Nielsen G.A., Schall M.W.: Developing strategies to spread improvements. In Joint Commission on Accreditation of Healthcare Organizations: *From Front Office to Front Line: Essential Issues for Health Care Leaders.* Oakbrook Terrace, IL: Joint Commission Resources, 2005, pp. 145–176.

8. Massoud M.R., et al.: *A Framework for Spread: From Local Improvements to System-Wide Change.* (IHI Innovation Series white paper.) Cambridge, MA: Institute for Healthcare Improvement, 2006.

9. Fraser S.W.: *Accelerating the Spread of Good Practice: A Workbook for Health Care.* West Sussex, UK: Kingsham Press, 2002.

10. Brown J.S., Duguid P.: *The Social Life of Information.* Boston: Harvard Business School Press, 2000.

11. Dixon N.: *Common Knowledge: How Companies Thrive by Sharing What They Know.* Boston: Harvard Business School Press, 2000.

12. Henderson D., et al.: Check a box. Save a life: How student leadership is shaking up health care and driving a revolution in patient safety. *J Patient Saf* 6:43–47, Mar. 2010.

CHAPTER 10

A Chapter for Educators: Designing Ways for Students to Learn to Improve Care

OBJECTIVES

After reading this chapter, you will be able to do the following:

1. Recognize the imperative for teaching health professionals in training about quality improvement.
2. Assess developmental levels when implementing quality improvement curricula.
3. Identify educational principles essential to developing learning experiences in quality improvement.
4. Describe examples of learning experiences in quality improvement.

"What I hear, I forget.
What I see, I remember.
What I do, I understand."
—*Confucius*

Jennifer Sorensen, an attending hospitalist in the internal medicine department, and Tomas Muñoz, a nurse educator working in a medical unit, are both excited. As coworkers in a medical unit of a major academic medical center, both find their jobs challenging and stimulating. Their focus is on caring for patients, but they also enjoy working with medical and nursing students who are eager to learn, who ask thought-provoking questions, and who contribute to patient care. Now Jennifer and Tomas have a new opportunity to provide high-quality care and teach at the same time: They have realized they can integrate the improvement of health care into the delivery and teaching of patient care.

As members of the hospital's rapid response team, Jennifer and Tomas saw improvement in action, with a one-third reduction in the hospital cardiac arrest rate since the team's implementation a year earlier. Patients who otherwise might have died were surviving and leaving the hospital. Jennifer and Tomas saw how working on improvement across professions makes it possible to provide better-individualized care, patient by patient. For example, thanks to the rapid response team protocol, a patient named Mrs. Jones was transferred into the intensive care unit much faster than she would have been in the old "call the ICU fellow" days. In addition, care has improved for an entire group of patients—people who, like Mrs. Jones, might otherwise have progressed to cardiac arrest.

Jennifer and Tomas decided that the ability to improve care needs to be part of what physicians and nurses learn from the very beginning of their education. They researched literature about education in quality improvement (QI) and grew more and more excited. Here was a place they could make a contribution! Some of the best minds in medicine and nursing agreed with them about the importance of teaching about improvement, but lots of questions remained about how best to do it. Should it be in the classroom? In the clinical setting, as part of rounds? Today Jennifer and Tomas are meeting with each other after speaking with the associate deans for curriculum of their respective schools. They had learned that the administrators at both schools were very enthusiastic and wanted faculty to lead this initiative. Now Jennifer and Tomas are wondering where to start.

Health Professional Development in the Improvement of Health Care Quality

In what will certainly become a classic editorial in the field of health care improvement, Batalden and Davidoff asked, "What is 'quality improvement' and how can it transform health care?"[1] They stated that QI is "the combined and unceasing efforts of everyone—health care professionals, patients and their families, researchers, payers, planners, educators—to make the changes that will lead to better patient outcomes (health), better system performance (care) and better professional development (learning)" (*see* Figure 10-1 on page 159).[1(p.2)] Jennifer and Tomas's experience on the rapid response team is an excellent example of these efforts.

In a follow-up to the landmark report *Crossing the Quality Chasm*,[2] the Institute of Medicine (IOM) convened an interprofessional panel to consider the implications for health professions education. The recommendations were published in 2003, in the *Health Professions Education: A Bridge to Quality* report:

> All students and working health professionals should develop and maintain proficiency in the following[3]:
> - Delivering patient-centered care
> - Working as part of interdisciplinary teams
> - Practicing evidence-based medicine
> - Focusing on QI
> - Using information technology

The Educational Imperative

Quality improvement is an increasingly visible aspect of clinical practice, but such work will not become "business as usual" until training in essential improvement skills is built into every level of health professional preparation. Fortunately, major educational and accrediting organizations across the health professions have begun to recognize this need.

FIGURE 10-1. *The Batalden and Davidoff "Triangle Diagram" to Demonstrate the Relationship of Everyone to the Three Core Pillars of Quality Improvement*

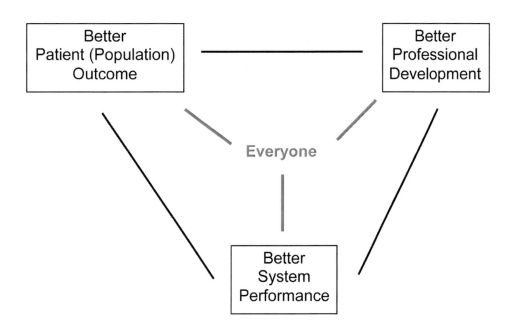

Source: Batalden P.B., Davidoff F.: What is "quality improvement" and how can it transform health care? *Qual Saf Health Care* 16:2–3, Feb. 2007. Adapted by permission from BMJ Publishing Group Limited.

Physician Training

Thought leaders in physician training have called for the incorporation of QI on two fronts:

1. The Association of American Medical Colleges (AAMC) recommended goals related to QI for medical students.[4]
2. The Accreditation Council for Graduate Medical Education (ACGME) included *practice-based learning and improvement* and *systems-based practice* as two of six core competencies for all resident physicians trained in the United States.[5]

In addition, the Carnegie Foundation Report *Educating Physicians: A Call for Reform of Medical School* recommended that "habits of inquiry and improvement" be incorporated into medical education by involving medical students and residents in QI efforts directed at the care of their patients.[6]

Nurse Training

Nursing education leaders believe there needs to be an increased QI presence in nursing curricula. According to a recent study, a large percentage of new nurses (39%) thought they were "poorly" or "very poorly" prepared about or had "never heard" of QI.[7] Nursing has worked to create a comprehensive response to the IOM recommendation across professional, accrediting, and educational organizations.

The American Association of Colleges of Nursing (AACN) and the American Nurses Association have endorsed QI as a core element of nurse education, and accreditation standards from accrediting bodies for nursing programs (such as the National League of Nursing Accrediting Center and Collegiate Commission on Nursing Education) are explicit about the necessity for the IOM competencies in all health in nursing prelicensure curricula. A 2010 report by the Carnegie Foundation for the Advancement of Teaching National Study of Nursing recommends a radical transformation of nursing education to effectively address the practice–education gap. The authors emphasize that both didactic and clinical educational models need to more fully reflect the current health care emphases on QI and patient safety.[8]

Quality and Safety Education for Nurses (QSEN). The 2003 IOM recommendations have had a far-reaching impact on nursing education through Quality and Safety Education for Nurses (QSEN), an initiative funded by the Robert Wood Johnson Foundation (RWJF). QSEN is a vibrant national initiative for nurses and nursing educators, and it offers resources for integrating IOM's recommendations into models of nursing education (prelicensure and graduate). A core group of nursing leaders examined IOM's five competencies and added safety as a sixth competency, thereby recognizing nurses' unique position to protect patient safety. These six competencies are the foundation of QSEN. With the goal of clarifying the competency definitions, QSEN's core faculty outlined the knowledge, skills, and attitudes (KSAs) appropriate for pre-licensure education for each of the six competencies.[9] These competencies and associated learning objectives are clearly listed on QSEN's Web site: http://www.qsen.org. With multiphase growth since 2005, QSEN has successfully achieved its mission to be a comprehensive resource for quality and safety education for nurses.

Other Clinician Training

In addition to medicine and nursing, other health care disciplines are making similar changes in their education programs. The National Commission on Certification of Physician Assistants (NCCPA), in collaboration with three other national physician assistant organizations, established competencies for practice that mirror ACGME competencies,[10] and the 2010 NCCPA accreditation standards require curriculum in "patient safety, QI, prevention of medical errors and risk management."[11] Likewise, the Accreditation Council for Pharmacy Education (ACPE) incorporates knowledge and skills for medication safety, QI, and work in interdisciplinary teams as part of its standards for pharmacy students.[12] Another example is the American Dental Association Council on Dental Accreditation's (ADA–DCA's) 2010 statement emphasizing the need to teach dental students to "deliver patient-centered care as members of an interdisciplinary team. . . . [where patient care will] emphasize evidence-based practice, quality improvement approaches, the application of technology and emerging information, and outcomes assessment."[13(p.12)]

In 2008 the Institute for Healthcare Improvement (IHI) launched the IHI Open School for Health Professions, with the goal of creating an interprofessional educational

---

A core group of nursing leaders examined IOM's five competencies and added safety as a sixth competency, thereby recognizing nurses' unique position to protect patient safety.

QSEN

http://www.qsen.org

---

community that gives students in nursing, health administration, medicine, pharmacy, dentistry, policy, and other health professions skills to become change agents in health care improvement. Recognizing that key topics such as patient safety and QI were lacking in traditional health professions education curricula, the IHI Open School designed a catalog of online courses—freely available to students, residents, and university faculty—in these and other critical topic areas. More than 20,000 students have completed the IHI Open School's online courses (available at http://app.ihi.org/lms/onlinelearning.aspx), which many university faculty have incorporated into their curricula. These courses have sparked widespread interest among practicing health professionals who are seeking training in the core topics that the courses promote.

The overlap and commonalities among these and other health professional organizations are striking. Although different health professions have organized their competencies and requirements in different ways (for example, ACGME focuses on practice-based learning and improvement and systems-based practice, while QSEN focuses on QI and safety), they each encompass the recommendations of the 2003 IOM report and create a framework for both educators and learners to use in developing professional competency.

Defining Competency in Quality Improvement

Why do many organizations use the term *competency*? Why not use *skills*—or even *domains of learning*? The term *competency* was chosen because it links stages of professional development with general models of adult learning. Although different individuals acquire and assimilate knowledge and skills in different ways, an appreciation of general developmental stages permits both learners and educators (including instructors, mentors, and coaches) to create and structure optimal learning experiences. In the 1970s Hubert Dreyfus and Stewart Dreyfus, focusing on chess players and pilots, described five stages (and characteristics) of skill development: novice, advanced beginner, competent, proficient, and expert.[14] Since health professionals are expected to achieve a level of competence by the end of training, clinical educators must understand the experience of learners in each of the Dreyfus stages. In the 1980s nursing theorist Patricia Benner used the Dreyfus stages to articulate levels of clinical growth and development in expert nurse clinicians.[15] Benner's work has been foundational in informing nurse educators about the development of expertise in nurses. Recent work in nursing has been done to stratify QSEN's learning objectives to acknowledge developing clinical competency.[16]

Developmental Levels

Results of a national Delphi study identified learning objectives for beginning, intermediate, and advanced levels of nurses' development.[16] The following developmental levels apply to medical students, nursing students, and members of an interprofessional QI team (*see* Table 10-1 on pages 163–164):

- **Novice:** At the novice level, learners attend to basic rules rather than to the real-world application of these rules. (In the spirit of *Dragnet*, novices want "just the facts.") Instructors, in turn, must make these rules the focus of their educational efforts. Knowledge at this level is free of context, and, as a result, learners' application of such rules may produce poor results in the real world.

> For example, students assigned to an interprofessional team learn about QI tools by carrying out specific assigned tasks, such as interviewing key stakeholders to validate a draft fishbone diagram.

- **Advanced beginner:** As a novice gains initial experience with real situations, he or she progresses to the advanced beginner level. Experience interacts with and contextualizes the rule itself, and the nature of the interaction becomes important. This work in context enhances basic knowledge.

> In our example, an advanced beginner interprofessional QI team reviews a Web site to review the hospital in which the team will be working. Two great resources for this are the Hospital Compare Web site (http://www.hospitalcompare.hhs.gov) and the Joint Commission's Quality Check® (http://www.qualitycheck.org). The team explores these Web sites to learn about the patient outcomes of the hospital in which it is working and to identify priorities for improving patient outcomes. The team applies Plan–Do–Study–Act (PDSA) concepts to initiate a QI project focusing on the identified priorities. In examining patterns and trends of QI data, the team is able to recognize the importance of variance in understanding QI process outcomes.

Hospital Compare
*http://www.hospital
compare.hhs.gov*

Quality Check®
http://www.qualitycheck.org

- **Competent:** As an advanced beginner gains further experience, the number and variation of elements in the situation can become overwhelming. Learners begin to appreciate, however, which elements of a situation require attention and which do not. The vast possibilities (of interpretation or action) can be narrowed to a manageable few. In addition, a deep emotional attachment to the task now develops. The successes, failures, joys, and disappointments matter on a much deeper level.

> To continue our example, the interprofessional QI team identifies patient outcomes that need to be improved and initiates PDSA cycles. The team trends outcomes from PDSA cycles, identifying variance and effective improvement strategies. Each team member's appreciation grows for the other members' expertise as the cycles unfold.

- **Proficient:** At the proficient level, a practitioner continues to scroll through a complete list of possibilities but does so with much greater speed. An element of efficiency now accompanies the skill. Individuals develop the capacity to step back and to see more clearly the problem that needs to be solved, though often the solution itself still requires active deliberation. Increased efficiency enables the practitioner to remove waste from the work by directly connecting knowledge and skill to the problem at hand.

TABLE 10-1.

Levels of Professional Development: Dreyfus, Benner, and Interprofessional QI Teams

Developmental Level	Dreyfus	Benner/Nursing	Interprofessional QI Team Examples
Novice	• Novice practitioners identify and use rules of thumb. • Novice practitioners attend to basic rules themselves rather than to real-world application of these rules.	• Novice nurses have little understanding of the contextual meaning of recently learned textbook concepts. • Novice nurses base what they do on principles.	• Novices assigned to an interprofessional team learn about QI tools by carrying out specific assigned tasks, such as interviewing key stakeholders to validate a draft fishbone diagram.
Advanced beginner	• Advanced beginner practitioners connect rules to the common aspects of a plan. • Advanced beginner practitioners' experience interacts with and contextualizes the rule itself, and the nature of the interaction becomes important.	• Advanced beginner nurses begin to recognize recurring components of the patient situation. • Advanced beginner nurses are learning to discriminate between normal and abnormal patient situations and establish priorities for what is important.	• Advanced beginners use the Hospital Compare (http://www.hospitalcompare.hhs.gov) and Quality Check (http://www.qualitycheck.org) Web sites to study the patient outcomes of the hospital in which they will be working and compare these to the hospital's stated QI goals. • After identifying local QI priorities, an advanced beginner works with an already-established QI team to perform a system analysis of a specific unit. • Advanced beginners observe care being delivered, create process models, and collect defined baseline data.
Competent	• Competent practitioners are able to plan an approach and execute the plan. • Competent practitioners begin to appreciate, based on varied experiences, which elements of a situation require attention and which do not. The vast possibilities (of interpretation or action) can be narrowed to a manageable few. In addition, a deep emotional attachment to the task now develops. The successes, failures, joys, and disappointments matter on a much deeper level.	• Competent nurses are more adept at anticipating future patient needs. Their plan of care development is based on current knowledge derived from an analytic consideration of the problem at hand. • Competent nurses can promote efficiency and organization. • Although competent nurses have a sense of mastery and are able to cope with a number of variables, they still lack the speed and flexibility of proficient nurses.	• A competent interprofessional QI team identifies patient outcomes that need improvement and identifies small tests of change. • A competent interprofessional QI team is comfortable writing an aim, analyzing measures, identifying changes, and testing changes using iterative PDSA cycles. • A competent interprofessional QI team trends outcomes from PDSA cycles, identifying variance and effective improvement strategies. • A competent interprofessional QI team appreciates each member's expertise as the cycles unfold.

(continued)

TABLE 10-1.

Levels of Professional Development: Dreyfus, Benner, and Interprofessional QI Teams

(continued)

Proficient	• Proficient practitioners regularly use evidence-based work and take waste out of that work. • Proficient practitioners continue to scroll through a complete list of possibilities, but they do so with much greater speed. An element of efficiency now accompanies the skill. Individuals develop the capacity to step back and to see more clearly the problem that needs to be solved, though often the solution itself still requires active deliberation. Increased efficiency enables the practitioner to remove waste from the work by directly connecting knowledge and skill to the problem at hand.	• Proficient nurses perceive situations as wholes rather than as aspects. • Proficient nurses know from experience what to expect in given situations and how to modify plans. • Proficient nurses discover that rather than having to analyze and calculate a plan, the plan simply presents itself. • Because of the vast body of experience, proficient nurses are able to zero in on the problem with very little thought. • Proficient nurses use maxims to practice. These are nuances of a situation, and Benner notes that to nurses at any of the other levels of skill acquisition, these maxims appear unintelligible because of their ambiguity.	• A proficient interprofessional QI team experiences QI work as a regular yet episodic element in practice. • There is a notable increase in interprofessional QI team efficiency because of the increased capability of the team members. • Members of a proficient interprofessional QI team clearly value QI work, understand and appreciate the contributions of other team members, and regularly use QI methods.
Expert	• Expert practitioners can use intuition where empirical knowledge does not yet exist. • Expert practitioners develop a vast repertoire of skills and a capacity for situational discrimination that are achievable only through experience. Tasks are performed on a more intuitive level, and essential problems are recognized and immediately addressed. Expert practitioners also learn to comfortably manage situations in which the rules do not apply.	• Expert nurses have an intuitive grasp based on extensive experience. Rules, guidelines, and maxims are no longer necessary for dealing with familiar situations. • Expert nurses are able to zero in on the problem, and performance becomes fluid, flexible, and highly proficient. • Expert nurses have difficulty explaining what they know because their tacit knowledge has become internalized.	• An expert interprofessional QI team continuously redesigns health care processes with an emphasis on patient outcomes. • An expert interprofessional QI team maximizes the use of each member's expertise and intuitively knows which member can best address which aspect of a task. • An expert interprofessional QI team does this work as part of their routine care processes. • An expert interprofessional QI team moves beyond just doing QI and actively seeks to develop and test new QI methods and interventions. • An expert interprofessional QI team regularly publishes and presents their findings.

Sources: Dreyfus H., Dreyfus S.: *Mind over Machine.* New York: The Free Press, 1986; Benner P.: From *Novice to Expert: Excellence and Power in Clinical Nursing Practice.* Upper Saddle River, NJ: Prentice-Hall, 1984.

> In our example, the proficient interprofessional team experiences QI work as a regular yet episodic element in its practice. The team uses evidence to formulate QI questions and identify the best data points. At the proficient level, there is a notable increase in team efficiency because of the increased capability of the team members. Members of the QI team clearly value QI work and appreciate the contributions of other team members.

- **Expert:** An expert develops a vast repertoire of skills and a capacity for situational discrimination that are achievable only through experience. Tasks are performed on a more intuitive level, and essential problems are recognized and immediately addressed. Expert practitioners also learn to comfortably manage situations in which the rules do not apply.

> So, to complete our example, the expert interprofessional QI team continuously redesigns health care processes with an emphasis on patient outcomes. The team maximizes the use of each member's expertise and intuitively knows which member can best address which aspect of a task. The team does this work as part of its routine care processes.

In adapting the developmental language of the Dreyfus model to the specific challenges of health professional training in QI, educators recognize that training is a process of ongoing growth and development. Acquisition of specific knowledge and skills is essential for all professionals, but terms such as *competent* and *proficient* direct our attention to practitioners' underlying capacity *to assimilate* and *apply* this knowledge and these skills, with increasing sophistication, in the work of health care and its improvement. Today's competent health professional trainee matures into tomorrow's proficient and expert practitioner, so QI competence must mature and develop along with other professional knowledge and skills.

Developing Competency in Quality Improvement

Health care improvement is not a "spectator sport" but a participant-driven implementation of specific knowledge and skills. It cannot be learned passively by sitting in a lecture, watching a DVD, attending a meeting, or visiting a Web site, although Web sites, didactic sessions, and other materials can play important roles in preparing learners. Improvement requires action, and learning about improvement must be action based. But what skills and knowledge are required at each stage in this learning process so that students in the health professions achieve competence in QI before entering practice? Let us more closely examine each stage in this professional development so that we can identify specific improvement-oriented educational strategies.

Initiating a Novice

Health professional students begin their training as novices of QI, and they benefit from exposure to generic "rules" of improvement. The IHI has identified eight domains of knowledge for improvement work (*see* Table 10-2 on page 166).[17] These domains serve as a valuable framework for introducing students to QI theory and practice and for fostering QI curriculum development among faculty. They have served well as a guide to core content and have been used in multiple venues.[5] From these domains, it is possible to derive a set of learning objectives appropriate for learners involved in an introductory learning experience about QI and patient safety.[18] Of course, even this useful framework may feel abstract to a novice who has minimal real-world experience. A bridge to such experience, in contexts familiar to the student, can bring improvement principles to life.

Students also bring "naïve" eyes to the study of health care processes, and their perspective is valuable to improvement teams that seek to describe existing health care processes. Involving students in specific aspects of improvement work enables them to contribute insights that might be missed by more senior clinicians who are immersed everyday in the (dys)functions of the health care system. For instance, a student following a patient being admitted to the hospital from the emergency department can describe the steps of that process from the patient's point of view, identifying areas

TABLE 10-2.

The Institute for Healthcare Improvement's Eight Knowledge Domains for the Improvement of Health Care

Domain	Description
1. Health care as a process and system	• The interdependent people (patients, families, eligible populations, caregivers), procedures, activities, and technologies of caregiving that come together to meet the need(s) of individuals and communities
2. Variation and measurement	• The use of measurement to understand the variation of performance in processes and systems of work • Improvement of the design and redesign of health care
3. Customer/ beneficiary knowledge	• Identification of the person, persons, or groups for whom health care is provided • Assessment of their needs and preferences • The relationship of the provided health care to those needs and preferences
4. Leading, following, and making changes in health care	• The methods and skills for making changes in complex organizations • The general and strategic management of people and the health care work they do (financing, information technology, daily caregiving)
5. Collaboration	• The knowledge, methods, and skills needed to work effectively in groups • The understanding and valuing of the perspectives and responsibilities of others • The capacity to foster the same in others
6. Social context and accountability	• An understanding of the social contexts (local, regional, national, global) of health care • The financial impact and costs of health care
7. Developing new, locally useful knowledge	• The recognition of the need for new knowledge in personal daily health and professional practice • The skill to develop new knowledge through empiric testing
8. Professional subject matter	• The health professional knowledge appropriate for a specific discipline • The ability to apply and connect health professional knowledge to all of the above • Core competencies published by professional boards, accrediting organizations, and other certifying entities

Source: Institute for Healthcare Improvement: *Eight Knowledge Domains for Health Professional Students.* http://www.ihi.org/offerings/IHIOpenSchool/resources/ Pages/Publications/EightKnowledgeDomainsForHealthProfessionStudents.aspx (accessed May 1, 2011). Reprinted from http://www.IHI.org with permission of the Institute for Healthcare Improvement.

for possible improvement. One study demonstrated that medical students reporting patient safety issues in an academic health center proposed interventions that were more robust than those suggested by health professionals in the center's patient safety reporting system.[19]

Developing Advanced Beginner Knowledge and Skills

An advanced beginner needs many opportunities to apply rules "in action." Such opportunities may be constructed around formal QI rotations or other hands-on experiences. These contexts also enable students to participate in (and to reap the benefits of) *interprofessional* learning, specifically through collaboration with learners across disciplines. Many professional schools and postgraduate education programs have developed integrated experiences that allow learners to simultaneously learn about QI and improve patient care on the front lines.

In the 2009–2010 academic year, the Josiah Macy Jr. Foundation and the IHI, through the IHI Open School, supported faculty teams from six universities as they developed curricula in QI and patient safety for medical and nursing students integrated into existing courses.[20] The faculty developed learning experiences in classrooms, simulation centers, and clinical settings. Overall there were 1,360 student encounters in 15 new learning activities, and 87% of them were interprofessional.

Ongoing Quality Improvement Competence for Clinicians

Developing competence (and proficiency or expertise) in QI is essential not only for students but also for practicing professionals. Practicing physicians will soon be expected to demonstrate competence in QI as part of their maintenance of certification. The American Board of Medical Specialties defines four components required for maintenance of certification, one of which is "Practice Performance Assessment." Physicians in all member specialties are asked to demonstrate that they can assess the quality of care they provide compared to peers and national benchmarks and then apply the best evidence or consensus recommendations to improve that care using follow-up assessments.[21] Because most postlicensure programs (like most undergraduate health professional education programs) provide only introductory knowledge and experience with improvement methods, adequate preparation for competent practitioners can be challenging to achieve. Faculty who are skilled and comfortable with teaching QI are still relatively limited in number.

Advanced QI competence. Some residency programs have significantly redesigned their teaching and practice structures and have developed specific learning experiences to prepare competent QI practitioners. The AAMC's Chronic Care Collaborative,[22] for example, was very successful in coordinating patient care and practice redesign with formal QI teaching. This collaboration across more than 20 medical centers resulted in many resident practices outperforming staff physician practices in outcomes for diabetes care. This is another example of how activities of patient care, practice improvement, and professional learning are interdependent and mutually supportive—particularly when thoughtful planning supports the integration.

QI competence and leadership. In another example, the Dartmouth-Hitchcock Leadership Preventive Medicine Residency (DHLPMR) program offers a new approach to preventive medicine training, linking it with the other clinical residencies offered at the institution and requiring a major leadership experience in QI for successful program completion.[23] DHLPMR residents have redesigned care for patients with pneumonia, improved care for hospitalized diabetic patients, increased the safety and efficacy of sedation for endoscopic procedures, and optimized use of electronic medical records to address obesity in a community health clinic. This leadership experience occupies two full years of residency, requires extensive coordination between academic and clinical settings, and enjoys significant support from senior leadership of the institution. Such commitment is possible because the program not only develops knowledge and skills in both residents and faculty but also stimulates tangible improvements in patient experience, clinical outcomes, and health system costs.

QI skill development in fellowship programs. Since 1999, the U.S. Department of Veterans Affairs (VA) Office of Academic Affiliations has sponsored a two-year postresidency fellowship for physicians, the VA National Quality Scholars Fellowship Program (NQSFP).[24] The NQSFP was created to develop academic, research, teaching, and administrative physician leaders in QI. In 2009 the NQSFP expanded to welcome doctoral-trained nurse fellows, making it the first interprofessional improvement fellowship in the world. Fellows and faculty work closely together to advance the scholarship of improvement. They focus on developing and testing novel teaching methods for nursing and medical students, researching new ways of delivering care, and sharing their work through peer-reviewed publications and presentations. More than 80 individuals have completed the program and have assumed leadership roles in health care institutions throughout the world.

QI competence for QSEN faculty. An important facet of QSEN's work has been faculty development. QSEN's Web site, http://www.qsen.org, was developed to be a rich resource for nursing faculty to educate themselves about updated quality and safety concepts and thus more competently teach QI. The site has an abundant supply of peer-reviewed teaching/learning activities for the classroom, clinical rotation, learning lab, and simulation that are ready for use. The site includes videos of landmark safety cases (for example, the Lewis Blackman and Josie King cases), as well as annotated bibliographies for QSEN's six competencies, which are updated every six months. Phase III support of QSEN by the Robert Wood Johnson Foundation for QSEN (2009–2012) included funding for eight regional workshops to educate nursing faculty about the current state of the science in health care quality and safety.

General Principles for Educational Experiences in Health Care Improvement

In the scenario at the beginning of this chapter, Jennifer and Tomas were excited about the opportunity to incorporate QI and patient safety into medical and nursing education. They asked themselves, "Where do we start?" The following four principles for building educational experiences in health care improvement help to answer that question. These principles apply at any developmental level. The first three echo what medical educators have found helpful when teaching in other content areas. The remaining principle reflects what is needed for successful change and improvement in health care.

Principle 1: The Learning Experience Should Be a Combination of Didactic and Project-Based Work

Like other complex clinical tasks, learning to improve health care requires mastering new content, acquiring new skills, and demonstrating appropriate attitudes. Thus there is a need for reading and discussion, reflection, practice, feedback, more discussion, more reflection, more reflection, and more feedback—the classic cycle of experiential learning described by Kolb.[25]

Many of us have learned this lesson the hard way—and sometimes more than once! One early course in improvement that included medical, nursing, and health administration students at Case Western Reserve University started out with a strong dose of theory, followed by interprofessional student group visits to local health care improvement teams.[26] Each student group's assignment was to learn about the team's project, interview the participants, and report on how what they'd observed illustrated the theory discussed in class. In their feedback about the course, the students strongly endorsed the connection to real-world health care improvement work, but like other health professional students, they wanted to participate, not just observe. (We know what you're thinking: This point does seem obvious now!) The next time the course was offered, interprofessional student teams worked on projects sponsored by local health care improvement leaders, usually carved out from a larger initiative. The course faculty prepared the students with several weeks of didactic work before the projects began. Student feedback was more positive than before, but the students felt strongly that they had to wait too long before getting to work on their projects.

By the time the course reached a steady-state model (with consistently high ratings from both the students and the project sponsors), the students signed up for their projects as part of signing up for the course, had their first student team meeting as part of the first class, and started on their projects right away. Didactic work in class was reorganized to support the project work, not the other way around. Student learning, as measured by the quality of project reports, improved. Project sponsors returned to offer student projects year after year. Even teams made up of novice health professional students contributed to health care improvement projects in ways that were valuable to the host organizations. This leads to two corollary principles:

1. Didactic learning seems to "stick" best when it is related to project work.
2. The most stimulating projects are those that are most likely to create direct benefit for patients.

All of this echoes what generations of students have said: that learning in the context of real patient problems is most stimulating and most likely to be retained over time.[27]

Principle 2: Link with Health System Improvement Efforts

A long-standing (and not yet resolved) controversy among health care improvement teachers is the value of learner-initiated improvement projects. The argument is compelling: Learners will be most stimulated to work on (and learn from) projects they have identified themselves, in which they have a particular interest. The problem is that what learners wish to improve may not align with the top priorities of health care organizations and their leaders. In that case, progress may occur as long as the student-champion keeps the work going. When the inevitable occurs and the student moves on to another course, another clerkship, another rotation, or another training program, work on the project may end. Much to the frustration of both students and faculty, this often happens before significant improvements have occurred—even with the best student efforts and ideas. A better approach is to align improvement learning with actual clinical projects.[28,29] We suggest two ways to deal with this dilemma: (1) Carefully prepare a learner-initiated project before the student gets started or (2) invite the student to choose from a menu of projects created from the list of current organizational priorities.

Carefully preparing a learner-initiated project before the student gets started. To prepare for a successful learner-initiated improvement project, it is important to ask who must support the work for anything new to happen. What part of the organization is involved? Who are the leaders? Whose support will be needed for progress to be made? Who will be the project champion (and team) after the student moves on? It is a good idea to talk with those people before any work starts and to enlist their help; ideally, you want to recruit them to be part of the improvement team. Consider the triangle in Figure 10-1: In any health care organization, improved patient outcomes and system performance will be as important as excellent professional development. Who needs to be involved, and what will it take to be sure that a learner-initiated project resonates in all three areas?

An example of preparation for a successful learner-initiated improvement project is a project done by a medical resident to decrease the rate of central line–associated infections in a medical intensive care unit (MICU) through more reliable use of full-barrier protection (that is, sterile drapes, gown, gloves, and mask) during line insertion. The resident was passionate about the project, but his success depended on partnerships with leaders in the MICU who had the authority to make things happen. In this case, a key partner was the nurse unit manager, who worked with the resident to test the interventions (including a procedure cart with all the necessary materials easily at hand) and to sustain their use over time (after the resident finished his part of the project and moved on to another rotation). Without these steps, learners may become very frustrated at not being able to get anything done or, even with a successful project, having no way to sustain improvements when the learners must inevitably personally move on to other assignments.

A common and widely used assignment for senior nursing students is to identify and execute a QI project during a cumulative clinical capstone course. Having students work closely with unit managers in identifying these projects creates mutual benefit for the senior nursing student and the nursing unit. The nursing literature is replete with examples of such projects.[30–32]

Inviting a student to choose from a menu of projects created from the list of current organizational priorities. An alternate approach to preparing for a successful learner-initiated improvement project is to identify health care improvement efforts that are already in place and thus already have gained the support and investment of the organization's leaders. It is often not difficult to identify a part of the work that could benefit from another set of willing hands. It is challenging to have students become part of project teams; the rhythm of a student's life usually does not match the work cycle of an ongoing improvement team. Despite the best intentions on all sides, a student may be able to make routinely scheduled meetings during some courses or rotations but not others. Therefore, if someone from a team is willing to act as a project sponsor, students can often take over a certain area (think of it as a "subproject"), work on it during the time available to meet prespecified goals, and then hand it back to the team. An example is an organizational effort to improve the care of patients with sickle cell disease. The team identified multiple issues that led to patients with severe sickle cell disease receiving most of their care in the emergency department. While the team worked on improving the organization's approach to managing pain with sickle cell crises, a student team worked to identify the barriers to clinic follow-up after a sickle cell patient was seen in the emergency room. The students interviewed the patients to understand the issues from the patients' point of view and made several recommendations that the team later tested.

Principle 3: Assess Education Outcomes

As part of an outstanding review of interprofessional education, Hugh Barr created a helpful elaboration of the classic Kirkpatrick model of education outcomes. We share it in Table 10-3 on page 172, along with an example of the model's application in improvement education.[33] This was published two years before Batalden and Davidoff's editorial (*see* Figure 10-1); the similarities are striking. Perhaps we shouldn't be surprised; after all, improvement work, at its core, is about learning. It is impressive

TABLE 10-3.
Barr-Kirkpatrick Hierarchy of Educational Outcomes

Education Outcome	Example
1. Reaction	End-of-experience student feedback
2a. Modification of attitudes/ perceptions	Pre and post student responses to written assessment of attitudes related to health care quality, patient safety, and interprofessional teamwork
2b. Acquisition of knowledge/skills	Assessment of ability to read a case scenario, identify an improvement need, write an aim statement, identify an appropriate measure, and propose a change to test
3. Behavioral change	During a clinical rotation, 360-degree assessment of behaviors consistent with collaboration and teamwork
4a. Change in organizational practice	Change in care as a result of an improvement initiative
4b. Benefits to patients/clients	Change in patient outcomes related to an improvement initiative

Source: Adapted from Barr H., et al.: *Effective Interprofessional Education: Argument, Assumption and Evidence.* Oxford, UK: Blackwell Publishing, 2005.

We suggest that teachers creating learning experiences in health care improvement focus on a few key outcome measures (perhaps one from each level of Barr's hierarchy, as far up as you can reach) and work to collect measures in a way that will give feedback to both the learners and the teachers.

that these experts identified change in organizational practice and benefits to patients as the highest order of education outcomes.

At the bottom of the scale is the most basic of education outcomes: learner feedback. Although important, learner feedback is insufficient to judge the quality of the experience. In fact, when used alone, learner feedback can be misleading. One recent effort found that medical residents who experienced (and liked) a popular classroom-based introduction to improvement performed no better than controls when their improvement learning was tested using a written knowledge application assessment.[34] In contrast, medical residents who underwent a course involving a combination of a health care improvement project and didactics performed much better than controls on a similar instrument.[28] Although both groups of residents rated their learning experiences highly, they performed much differently when their ability to apply what they learned was assessed.

Education about QI in health care creates opportunities for educators to link their efforts to improvements in patient outcomes and organizational performance, the top of Barr's outcomes hierarchy. Some have succeeded in doing just that, even with inexperienced learners.[19,29,35] We suggest that teachers creating learning experiences in health care improvement focus on a few key outcome measures (perhaps one from each level of Barr's hierarchy, as far up as you can reach) and work to collect measures in a way that will give feedback to both the learners and the teachers. A helpful question might be "What is the single most important attribute I'm trying to engender in these learners? How can I measure that in a way that will be useful?"

Principle 4: Model QI in Educational Processes
The education outcomes described in the preceding sections have a dual purpose: feedback for the learner and feedback for the teacher. We believe that part of the work of teaching improvement is modeling the same improvement behaviors in our work as

educators. Why would students believe that QI is important if they don't see faculty improving their own work, both as clinicians and educators?

In the examples described in the preceding sections, the faculty got important information about educational outcomes through surveys to collect learner feedback, written tests of learner ability to apply knowledge, structured assessments of student team project reports, organization sponsor feedback, and changes in organizational practice and patient outcomes. Any and all of these can be used to improve a course over time, applying QI to the education experience itself. But faculty need to be sure to schedule time to reflect on the results and make decisions about the future. When the teaching is over and the student feedback is given, it is easy to move on to the next agenda item in our busy professional lives. Quality improvement depends on reflection (the act phase of the PDSA cycle described in Chapter 8), without which our efforts will fail to improve over time.

The ACGME mandate. In July 2006 the ACGME Outcome Project moved into its third phase, requiring graduate medical education programs to demonstrate their use of resident outcomes for program improvement. Such demonstration requires that programs know the needs of the residents they are educating, understand their own training processes and patterns, define measures related to educational outcomes, collect data on those outcomes, and develop ways to improve the training processes that result in improved outcomes. In other words, residency program directors must use QI knowledge and skills on their own programs! While this mandate represents a challenge to program directors, who must endeavor to learn more about their own educational processes and outcomes (including patient care outcomes), it also provides both faculty and residents with new opportunities to teach and to learn the methods of QI.

Summary

Let's return to the opening scenario. Jennifer Sorensen, the hospitalist, and Tomas Muñoz, the nurse educator, are right: There is still a lot to learn about teaching health professional students about the improvement of health care. In addition to becoming education leaders at their schools, Jennifer and Tomas can study the education innovations they create and publish scholarly work that would advance the field.

Examples of Improvement Curriculum and Resources

In a review published in 2003, Ogrinc et al. presented a matrix of learning objectives in the eight IHI domains of improvement knowledge matched to the level of learner— beginning medical student (novice) through advanced resident (competent).[36] This developmental approach prompted specific examples of teaching strategies at each level. (*See* Table 10-4 on pages 174–175 for an adapted table that includes both nursing and medical learners.) Note that there is an attempt to focus improvement learning (and work) on areas familiar to the learner, from education itself (for beginning students) to the systems of care for groups of patients (for advanced

TABLE 10-4.

Examples of Teaching Strategies, by Level of Learners[36]

Learner Level	Examples of Medical Teaching Strategies	Examples of Nursing Teaching Strategies
Beginning prelicensure learner (novice)	In large-group lecture format, medical students learn the basics of clinical improvement sciences, health care systems, and an introduction to population and improvement statistical methods. Through small-group sessions, medical students focus on health care systems. Collaborating with other students, they will (1) develop an aim and an understanding of the process, (2) measure process or outcome variables, and (3) try a test of change (PDSA cycle) on a system that is important to them (such as a study group). Projects are summarized and presented to the entire class.	Faculty and students review the elements of rapid-cycle improvement processes used for QI work in health care. Nursing students read Atul Gawande's article "The Checklist" from the December 2007 *New Yorker* as an example of effective QI work that significantly improved patient outcomes, available on Atul Gawande's Web site (http://www.gawande.com) and write a reflection on the role of nurses in Dr. Pronovost's work. Nursing students review central-line policies at the hospital where they are currently doing a clinical rotation and analyze how they compare with standards for central-line placement and maintenance.
Advanced prelicensure learner (advanced beginner)	Medical students convene in small groups to focus on a clinical improvement project that is ongoing within an affiliated health care facility. With guidance from the clinical QI team, students focus on a distinct patient group (such as sickle cell disease, congestive heart failure, asthma). The group will (1) develop an aim; (2) describe how various disciplines work together to form the system of care for these patients; (3) identify, collect, and display appropriate measures of care, including cost; and (4) recommend changes that the clinical improvement team might test. Summarized reports are presented to the organization's clinical improvement leaders.	As part of their perioperative rotation, nursing students examine QI in the surgical setting. They review the Surgical Care Improvement Project (SCIP) that is integrated into the Centers for Medicare & Medicaid Services (CMS) and The Joint Commission's core measures. Students go to The Joint Commission's website (http://www.jointcommission.org) and review the elements of the SCIP core measure. They track where they are seeing the elements of the SCIP core measure implemented in the clinical setting and identify which elements are the responsibility of nursing. Students interview a perioperative nurse manager and inquire about current QI projects in preop, the operating room, or the postanesthesia care unit. What data are being collected for these projects? Which patient outcome will this QI work improve? How is rapid-cycle change process being used? Students present their observations about the SCIP core measure and current QI projects to their clinical group.
Beginning postlicensure learner (competent)	With mentoring from faculty members, a medical resident focuses on his or her own emerging practice. After conducting an assessment of his or her patients' needs, an aim is specified to address those needs. By the resident's engaging other members of the health care team—ideally from various disciplines—the process of care is mapped, and balanced measures are explored to follow the process. Small tests of change are initiated to improve care.	With mentoring from faculty, new graduate nurse residents identify which quality indicators are being tracked at the facility where they are doing their cumulative capstone clinical rotations. They identify a problematic patient outcome at this facility (using http://www.hospitalcompare.hhs.gov). The nurses decide how they will collect baseline data and compare the local situation to national quality standards and initiatives. The nurses plot out the QI process: Which quality tools to use? What information is needed to guide changes? How might these data be collected? Working with other health professionals on the unit, the nurses conduct a small test of change. They review the results and share what they learned with the faculty. They plan and conduct a second small test of change. After analyzing data from the two PDSA cycles, the nurses summarize and present all parts of this process, the findings and experience.

(continued)

TABLE 10-4.

Examples of Teaching Strategies, by Level of Learners *(continued)*

Learner Level	Examples of Medical Teaching Strategies	Examples of Nursing Teaching Strategies
Advanced postlicensure learner (proficient)	Advanced clinicians continually monitor the system of care to observe how it reacts to changes. Because changes and improvements are ongoing, reassessment of patient needs may be necessary. The balanced instrument panel is modified as needed. Extending the improvement effort to other patient groups or other settings is encouraged, as is accessing community resources for the patients. Advanced clinicians also mentor the beginning clinician through improvement efforts. The improvement efforts may form the basis for grand rounds presentations and may be used to fulfill a research requirement.	A proficient nurse targets a Hospital Consumer Assessment of Healthcare Providers and Systems patient outcome on his or her nursing unit that has been evaluated as lower than national or local benchmarks. This registered nurse may choose process of care measures or outcome of care measures as his or her focus. Gathering resources from national initiatives, this registered nurse leads a staff team to improve targeted outcomes. This nurse leader may also use this project to mentor prelicensure students in the improvement process. Results are implemented on the unit, presented at grand nursing rounds, and standardized to influence evidence-based nursing policies in the hospital or health care system.

Source: Adapted from Ogrinc G., et al.: A framework for teaching medical students and residents about practice-based learning and improvement, synthesized from a literature review. *Acad Med* 78:748–756, Jul. 2003.

clinicians). With school curricula increasingly emphasizing early clinical experiences, there are many examples in which even beginning medical and nursing students have contributed to improvement work in health and health care.[29,37-42]

A Medical School Example

The School of Medicine at the University of Missouri in Columbia, Missouri, is an example of a medical school working to build a continuum of learning about improvement in health care. In fact, "committed to improving quality and safety in health care" is one of eight key characteristics that the school is working to achieve for its graduates. Table 10-5 on page 176 summarizes the work so far. An important strategy has been to integrate improvement learning as part of already-occurring educational activities, from a fourth-year medical student talk at the white coat ceremony to improvement work as part of an interprofessional team in the fourth year. Students are asked to provide evidence of their improvement work as part of their medical student portfolios. This creates an opportunity for assessing the development of these skills across courses and over the four years of the curriculum. Significant efforts, such as meaningful contributions to a clinical improvement team, can be included as part of the Medical School Performance Evaluation (formerly known as the "Dean's Letter") for residency applications.

The QSEN Model

As described on page 160 earlier in this chapter, QSEN is a national leader in paving the way to integrate QI into nursing curricula. The QSEN Web site, http://www.qsen.org, offers outstanding peer-reviewed teaching/learning strategies that have been adopted by many nursing programs.

TABLE 10-5.

A Continuum of Learning About the Improvement of Health Care at the University of Missouri (MU) School of Medicine

Medical School Year	Curricular Element	Description	Outcomes
1	White coat ceremony (required)	Review of key characteristics of MU grads, including the ability to deliver effective patient-centered care, the ability to collaborate with patients and other members of the health care team, and a commitment to improving quality and safety. Illustrated with reflections from a fourth-year medical student on what these meant in the context of a patient's story.	This addition to the white coat ceremony introduced in 2004. Very popular among first-year medical students and their families, so repeated yearly since.
1	Partners in Education–Partners in Care series in Introduction to Patient Care course	Longitudinal series of interprofessional small-group sessions with students in accelerated nursing program. In 2010–2011, sessions included Interprofessional Teamwork & Communication, Introduction to Quality and Safety, Health Literacy, Culturally Sensitive Interviewing, and Health Ethics.	Content from these sessions included in course examinations.
1	Summer externship in patient safety (elective)	Six summer externships in office of clinical effectiveness, conducting patient safety research.	Each student produces a final product appropriate to the project. Some have led to abstracts at peer reviewed national meetings.
2	Interprofessional curriculum (required as part of Introduction to Patient Care course)	Four-week problem-based curriculum involving medical, nursing, respiratory therapy, pharmacy, and health management students. Student teams analyze an adverse event and propose improvements. Simulation experience on teamwork, patient safety, and patient-centered care added in 2009.	Many attitudes regarding patient safety and QI improved posttraining. Students' self-perception of safety skills improved. Students report increased knowledge of other professions and greater awareness of the importance of teamwork.[43,44]
3	Patient safety internal medicine conferences (required)	Two one-hour sessions imbedded within internal medicine third-year clerkship. At second session, students report safety issues they have observed while on clerkship, as well as proposed innovations to improve safety. Faculty members from school of medicine and health care system facilitate discussion.	Students report increased comfort in analyzing cause of an error and increased reporting of safety issues to supervising faculty following this conference.[19]
3	The Integrated Patient Safety (TIPS) curriculum (required as part of internal medicine clerkship)	Collaboration with School of Nursing funded by Institute for Healthcare Improvement and Macy Foundation. Dyads of medical and nursing students learn about patient safety and perform a falls risk assessment on a hospitalized patient.	Begun in fall 2009. Improved student confidence in assessing falls risk and positive patient response. Student-collected data reported to health system falls prevention team.[45]
4	Achieving Competence Today Curriculum (elective: 17 medical students participated in 2008–2009; 14 in 2009–2010; 19 in 2010–2011)	Fourth-year students are embedded within interprofessional QI teams consisting of other learners (including residents) and staff of MU Health Care. Just-in-time QI training provided to teams by interprofessional faculty team.	Enhanced QI knowledge compared to matched controls as measured by QI knowledge assessment tool. End-of-course presentations to system leaders regarding improvements made.[29]
4	One-Month Elective in Quality/Safety	One-month elective in the office of clinical effectiveness, working on a QI or patient safety project.	Each student produces a final product appropriate to the project.

Source: Table updated from Headrick L.A., et al.: University of Missouri School of Medicine in Columbia. *Acad Med* 85(suppl. 9):S310–S315, Sep. 2010.

Resources

The following resources are helpful for learning more about teaching QI. In particular, we recommend the Academy for Healthcare Improvement (AHI), a professional home for faculty and others who wish to advance the scholarly and educational foundation of QI in health care. The AHI Web site (http://www.A4HI.org) lists resources, including peer-reviewed curricular material, for professionals who want to teach about improvement. Members can submit their work for peer review; materials that are posted can be listed as scholarly products.

The following are also helpful resources:

- **The Accreditation Council for Graduate Medical Education (ACGME) Outcome Project (http://www.acgme.org/acWebsite/irc/irc_compIntro.asp):** The ACGME describes "practice-based learning and improvement" and "systems-based practice" as two of six core physician competencies. The ACGME Outcome Project has developed teaching and assessment strategies for these competencies.
- **The Centre for the Advancement of Interprofessional Education (CAIPE; http://www.caipe.org.uk) Promoting Partnership for Health:** This series is composed of three books that provide an outstanding review of interprofessional education:
  - Freeth D., et al.: *Effective Interprofessional Education—Development, Delivery and Evaluation.* Oxford, UK: Blackwell Publishing, 2005.
  - Barr H., et al.: *Effective Interprofessional Education: Argument, Assumption and Evidence.* Oxford, UK: Blackwell Publishing, 2005.
  - Meads G., et al.: *The Case for Interprofessional Collaboration.* Oxford, UK: Blackwell Publishing, 2005.
- **Langley et al.'s *The Improvement Guide*[46]:** This book is an excellent overview of improvement principles and methods. Even though this book is not written only for health care, we have used it successfully as a basic reference for medical students and physicians at all levels of training.
- **Quality and Safety Education for Nurses (QSEN; http://www.qsen.org):** Described earlier in this chapter, the QSEN initiative maintains an active Web site that includes an annotated bibliography and a host of teaching strategies shared by educators from across the United States.

References

1. Batalden P.B., Davidoff F.: What is "quality improvement" and how can it transform health care? *Qual Saf Health Care* 16:2–3, Feb. 2007.

2. Committee on Quality of Health Care in America, Institute of Medicine: *Crossing the Quality Chasm: A New Health System for the 21st Century.* Washington, DC: National Academy Press, 2001.

3. Greiner A.C., Knebel E. (eds.): *Health Professions Education: A Bridge to Quality.* Washington, DC: National Academies Press, 2003.

4. Batalden P.B.: *Report V: Contemporary Issues in Medicine: Quality of Care.* Washington DC: Association of American Medical Colleges, Aug. 2001.

5. Leach D.C.: Evaluation of competency: An ACGME perspective. *Am J Phys Med Rehabil* 79:487–489, Sep.–Oct. 2000.

6. Cooke M., Irby D.M., O'Brien B.C.: *Educating Physicians: A Call for Reform of Medical School and Residency.* San Francisco: Jossey-Bass, 2010.

7. Kovner C.T., et al.: New nurses' views of quality improvement education. *Jt Comm J Qual Patient Saf* 36:29–35, Jan. 2010.

8. Benner P., et al.: *Educating Nurses: A Call for Radical Transformation.* San Francisco: Jossey-Bass, 2010.

9. Cronenwett L., et al.: Quality and safety education for nurses. *Nurs Outlook* 55:122–131, May–Jun. 2007.

10. National Commission on Certification of Physicians Assistants: *Physician Assistant Competencies: Online Center.* http://www.nccpa.net/PAC/Competencies_home.aspx (accessed May 1, 2011).

11. Accreditation Review Commission on Education for the Physician Assistant: *Accreditation Standards for Physician Assistant Education,* Mar. 2010. http://www.arc-pa.org/documents/Standards4theditionFINALwithclarifyingchangesJuly2010.pdf (accessed Oct. 12, 2011).

12. Accreditation Council for Pharmacy Education: *Accreditation Standards and Guidelines.* Jan. 23, 2011. http://www.acpe-accredit.org/standards/default.asp (accessed May 1, 2011).

13. American Dental Association Commission on Dental Accreditation: *Accreditation Standards for Dental Education Programs.* Aug. 6, 2010. http://www.ada.org/sections/educationAndCareers/pdfs/predoc.pdf (accessed May 1, 2011).

14. Dreyfus H., Dreyfus S.: *Mind over Machine.* New York: The Free Press, 1986.

15. Benner P.: From *Novice to Expert: Excellence and Power in Clinical Nursing Practice.* Upper Saddle River, NJ: Prentice-Hall, 1984.

16. Barton A.J., et al.: A national Delphi to determine developmental progression of quality and safety competencies in nursing education. *Nurs Outlook* 57:313–322, Nov.–Dec. 2009.

17. Batalden P., et al.: *Knowledge Domains for Health Professional Students Seeking Competency in the Continual Improvement and Innovation of Health Care.* Cambridge, MA: Institute for Healthcare Improvement, 1998.

18. Boonyasai R.T., et al.: Effectiveness of teaching quality improvement to clinicians: A systematic review. *JAMA* 298:1059–1061, Sep. 2007.

19. Hall L.W., et al.: Effectiveness of patient safety training in equipping medical students to recognise safety hazards and propose robust interventions. *Qual Saf Health Care* 19:3–8, Feb. 2010.

20. Headrick L.A., et al.: *Retooling for Quality and Safety: Integrating Quality and Safety into the Required Curriculum at Twelve Medical and Nursing Schools.* Manuscript under review.

21. American Board of Medical Specialties: *About ABMS Maintenance of Certification.* http://www.abms.org/About_Board_Certification/MOC.aspx (accessed May 1, 2011).

22. Association of American Medical Colleges Chronic Care Collaborative. Mar. 2008. https://www.aamc.org/download/70254/data/mar2008.pdf (accessed Oct. 18, 2011).

23. Foster T., et al.: Residency education, preventive medicine and population health care improvement: The Dartmouth-Hitchcock Leadership Preventive Medicine Approach. *Acad Med* 83:390–398, Apr. 2008.

24. Splaine M.E., et al.: The Department of Veterans Affairs National Quality Scholars Fellowship Program: Experience from 10 years of training quality scholars. *Acad Med* 84:1741–1748, Dec. 2008.

25. Kolb D.A.: *Experiential Learning: Experience as the Source of Learning and Development.* Upper Saddle River, NJ: Prentice-Hall, 1984.

26. Moore S., et al.: Using learning cycles to build an interdisciplinary curriculum in CI for health professions students in Cleveland. *Jt Comm J Qual Improv* 22:165–171, Mar. 1996.

27. Hoffman K., et al.: Problem-based learning outcomes: Ten years of experience at the University of Missouri–Columbia School of Medicine. *Acad Med* 81:617–625, Jul. 2006.

28. Ogrinc G., et al.: Teaching and assessing resident competence in practice-based learning and improvement. *J Gen Intern Med* 19:496–500, Mar. 2004.

29. Hall L.W., et al.: Linking health professional learners and health care workers on action-based improvement teams. *Qual Manag Health Care* 18:194–201, Jul.–Sep. 2009.

30. Christiansen A., Robson L., Griffith-Evans C.: Creating an improvement culture for enhanced patient safety: Service improvement learning in pre-registration education. *J Nurs Manag* 18:782–788, Oct. 2010.

31. Sherrod R.A., Morrison R.S.: Leadership experiences for baccalaureate nursing students: Improving quality in a nurse-managed rural health clinic. *Nurs Educ Perspect* 29:212–216, Jul.–Aug. 2008.

32. Bonner A., et al.: A student-led demonstration project on fall prevention in a long-term care facility. *Geriatr Nurs* 28:312–318, Sep.–Oct. 2007.

33. Barr H., et al.: *Effective Interprofessional Education: Argument, Assumption and Evidence.* Oxford, UK: Blackwell Publishing, 2005.

34. Morrison L.J., Headrick L.A.: Teaching residents about practice-based learning and improvement. *Jt Comm J Qual Patient Saf* 34:453–459, Aug. 2008.

35. Gould B.E., et al.: Improving patient care outcomes by teaching quality improvement to medical students in community-based practices. *Acad Med* 77:1011–1018, Oct. 2002.

36. Ogrinc G., et al.: A framework for teaching medical students and residents about practice-based learning and improvement, synthesized from a literature review. *Acad Med* 78:748–756, Jul. 2003.

37. Balestreire J.J., et al.: Teams in a community setting: The AUHS experience. *Qual Manag Health Care* 6:31–37, Winter 1998.

38. Chessman A.W., et al.: Students add value to learning organizations: The Medical University of South Carolina Experience. *Qual Manag Health Care* 6:38–43, Winter 1998.

39. Headrick L.A., et al.: Using PDSA (Plan-Do-Study-Act) to establish academic–community partnerships: The Cleveland Experience. *Qual Manag Health Care* 6:12–20, Winter 1998.

40. Horak B.J., O'Leary K.C., Carlson L.: Preparing health care professionals for quality improvement: The George Washington University/George Mason University experience. *Qual Manag Health Care* 6:21–30, Winter 1998.

41. Tschannen D., Aebersold M.: Improving student critical thinking skills through a root cause analysis pilot project. *J Nurs Educ* 49:475–478, Aug. 2010.

42. Thornlow D.K., McGuinn K.: A necessary sea change for nurse faculty development: Spotlight on quality and safety. *J Prof Nurs* 26:71–81, Mar. 2010.

43. Madigosky W.S., et al.: Changing and sustaining medical students' knowledge, skills, and attitudes about patient safety and medical fallibility. *Acad Med* 81:94–101, Jan. 2006.

44. Dyer C., et al.: *Integrating High Fidelity Simulation and Interprofessional Education in Patient Safety and Teamwork.* Academy for Healthcare Improvement Scientific Symposium, Orlando, Dec. 2009. http://www.a4hi.org/symposium/2009/abstracts/2Dyer.pdf (accessed Oct. 12, 2011).

45. Dyer C., et al.: *Using Fall Prevention for Interprofessional Patient Safety Training at the Bedside.* Academy for Healthcare Improvement Scientific Symposium. Orlando, Dec. 2010. https://www.aamc.org/download/249618/data/2011iqdyer.pdf (accessed Oct. 12, 2011).

46. Langley G.J., et al.: *The Improvement Guide: A Practical Approach to Enhancing Organizational Performance*, 2nd ed. San Francisco: Jossey-Bass, 2009.

Index

A

Academy for Healthcare Improvement (AHI), 177

Accountability measurement, 82

Accreditation Council for Graduate Medical Education (ACGME), 159, 173, 177

Accreditation Council for Pharmacy Education (ACPE), 160

Adaptable elements, 125, 127

Advanced beginner level, 162, 163, 167

Advanced postlicensure learner, 175

Advanced prelicensure learner, 174

Agency for Healthcare Research and Quality (AHRQ), 38–39

Aim statement
  creating, 50–51
  examples of, 51–52
  S.M.A.R.T. criteria for, 51
  theoretical limit for, 45

American Association of Colleges of Nursing (AACN), 160

American Association of Medical Colleges (AAMC) Chronic Care Collaborative, 167

American Board of Medical Specialties, 167

American Dental Association Council on Dental Accreditation (ADA–DCA), 160

American Nurses Association, 160

Anesthesia cards, 78

Assignable variation. *See* Special cause variation

Association of American Medical Colleges (AAMC), 49, 159

Authority gradients, 37

B

Background questions
  answers to, 21
  vs. clinical experience, 20
  description of, 19
  finding evidence with, 21

BAMI team. *See also* Improvement team
  aim of, 11
  brainstorming sessions by, 11
  worksheet, 12

Barr, Hugh, 171

Batalden, Paul, 84

Batalden and Davidoff "Triangle Diagram," 8, 159

Bayside Medical Center (BMC), 128, 136, 142

Beginning postlicensure learner, 174

Beginning prelicensure learner, 174

Benner, Patricia, 161

Berwick, Donald, 83

Beta-blocker after myocardial infarction (BAMI) team. *See* BAMI team

Beta-blocker usage
  explanation for differences in, 3, 5
  for heart failure, 98
  at individual hospitals, 5
  for Medicare patients, 4
  Model for Improvement for, 10–12
  for myocardial infarction, 2–3